All Is Well

The Art {and Science} of Personal Well-Being

The Covid Edition

All Is Well

The Art {and Science} of Personal Well-Being

2nd edition
The Covid edition

Marilynn Preston

Creators Publishing
Hermosa Beach, CA

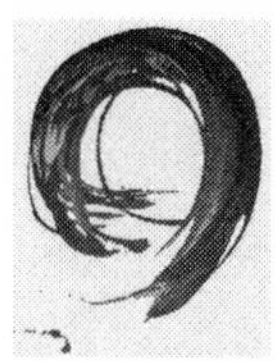

The enso contains the perfect and imperfect;
that is why it's always complete.
—Kazuaki Tanahashi

All Is Well

The Art {and Science} of Personal Well-Being

Cover design by Peggy Pfeiffer
Cover art courtesy of Kazuaki Tanahashi
Back cover author photo by Clara Lu
Winter, Spring, Summer, Autumn photos by Barbara Bonfigli
Additional photos by Karuna Tanahashi and Catriona McIlwraith
Creative Coordinators: Kelly Evans and Alessandra Caruso

CREATORS PUBLISHING
737 3rd St.
Hermosa Beach, CA 90254
A Blue Zone community

310-337-7003

LIBRARY OF CONGRESS CONTROL NUMBER: 2021950925

ISBN (PRINT): 978-1-949673-63-0

ISBN (EBOOK): 978-1-949673-62-3

SECOND EDITION

PRINTED IN THE UNITED STATES OF AMERICA

3 5 7 9 10 8 6 4

In gratitude to my readers. Without you, nothing.

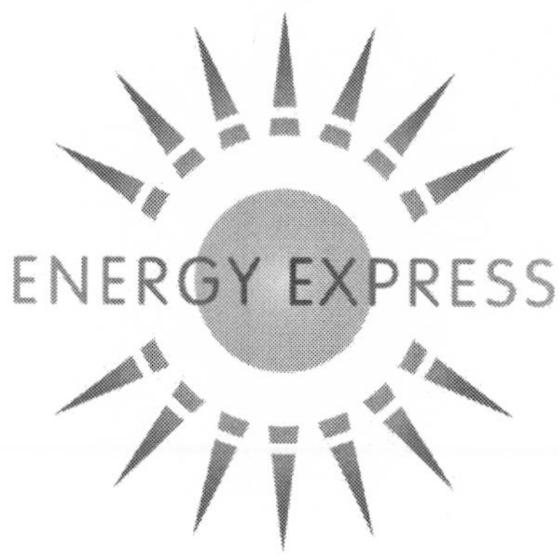

Tell me, what is it you plan to do
with your one wild and precious life?
—Mary Oliver

Table of Contents

Summer

Autumn

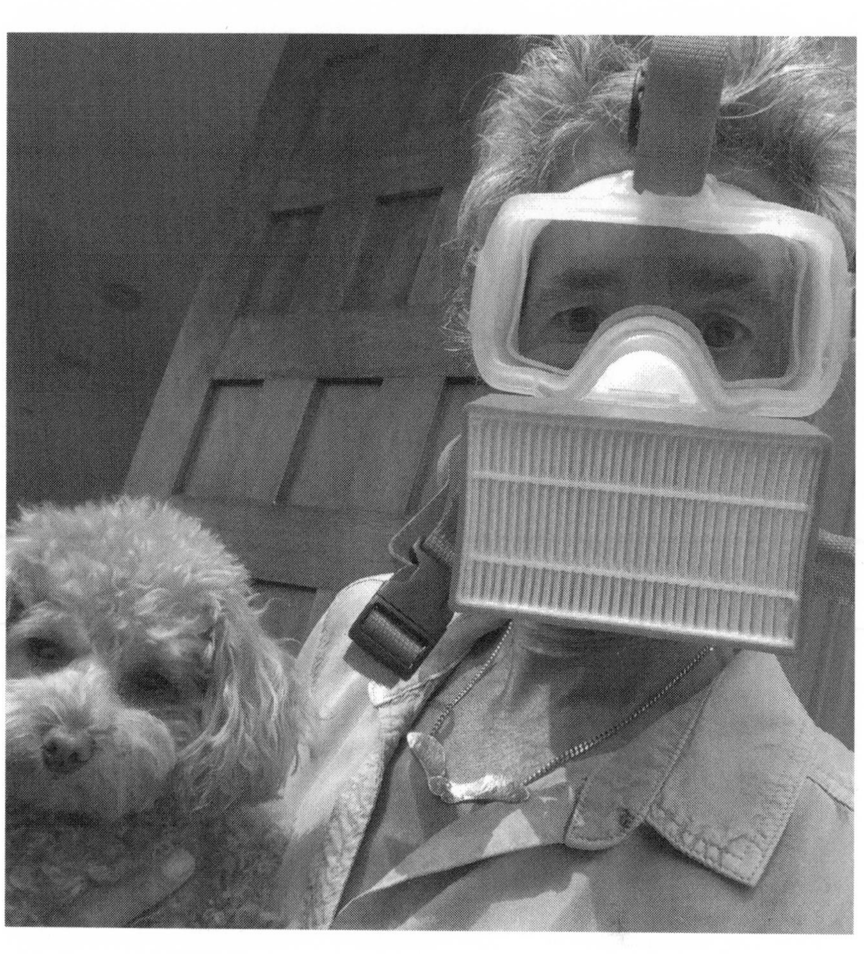

From the Author.

About six months into the COVID-19 global pandemic—after *My Brilliant Friend* but before *Schitt's Creek*—I realized I wanted to write a second edition of this book.

A few weeks after that—just before my second Zoom drumming lesson—I was talking on the phone to my publisher at Creators, and Jack asked if I was interested in writing a second edition. I took it as a sign, a happy coincidence, unlike the pandemic, a singular plunge into boundless suffering.

And now, here it is, the COVID edition, a deeper, darker, more demanding version of *All Is Well: The Art {and Science} of Personal Well-Being.* (But still a fun read.)

Why deeper? Because the COVID-19 pandemic was an apocalyptic wake-up call for all of us. It made me want to dig ever so much more into what it takes to evolve into a healthier and happier human, especially when the world as we know it is collapsing and transforming around us.

Why darker? Because 2020 was a humbling and horrifying year, and there is still so much grief and heartache, uncertainty and fear. Of course, there's light at the end of the tunnel. It's helping you find the light *inside* the tunnel that made me want to write a second edition.

And this edition is more demanding, dear reader, because the evidence is clearer than ever: Your personal well-being depends on you, the choices you make, and your willingness to take care of yourself and others in the kindest and best possible way. I know I told you that in the first edition, but this time, I really mean it.

So, to kick off this second edition, I want to share a few of my favorite lessons learned from the global pandemic, six powerful "aha! insights" I had while waiting for the world to return to normal, which it never will.

1. I learned that better breathing saves lives...starting with mine. Don't turn up your nose. This is serious. I'm convinced that learning about the power of nasal breathing saved my life during COVID. Let me explain.

I'd had a diagnosis of atypical pneumonia in late October 2019, a few months before the wicked and novel coronavirus put our country on pause.

I was as sick as I've ever been in my life—high fever, deep fatigue, hysterical coughing, drowning in mucus every morning—and thanks to the right combination of drugs by my doctor, I recovered. When I went into lockdown in March 2020, I knew my lungs were super vulnerable. I was scared.

But it wasn't just *learning* about nasal breathing that calmed my fears, strengthened my lungs, and helped heal my respiratory system. It was actually *doing* the nasal breathing, practicing my exercises many mornings and during the afternoon, too, when I could remember, which wasn't all that often.

I also signed up for a life-changing Breathing as Medicine course, a six-week, science-based intensive class with the very intense breathing master Ed Harrold. It was amazing.

I also doubled down on my yoga and studied more nasal breathing techniques—called pranayama—with my trusted yoga teachers Tias Little, Sienna Smith, Jo Lewzey, Nathan James, and Sarah Steen.

Patrick McKeown—who teaches Buteyko breathing on YouTube—was a big influence, as was his book *The Oxygen Advantage.* And not only did I read James Nestor's bestselling book *Breath* three times, but I loved it so much I've given away fifteen copies to family and friends. They've all thanked me.

And what exactly is nasal breathing, you wonder? See? That's what's still making me crazy. I learned most people have no awareness of the importance of nasal breathing, including doctors I spoke with, including pulmonologists. If you drill down, lung specialists know it's a good idea, but it's not what they talk about to the public or patients, and it's certainly not Western medicine's standard of care.

Well, it is for me. And I'll tell you why in the second edition's new chapter called "Be a Mouth Taper." You can skip there now, if you want, but please come back.

Summing up, I would say learning to breathe in and out of my nose, not my mouth, was the most important thing I learned in 2020. In fact, it became an obsession, unlike my drumming lessons.

2. I learned how important it is to write stuff down, day to day, during a crisis like COVID because it's so easy to lose track of what you're doing and why you're doing it. Before you know it, the days disappear, and you've forgotten the basics of personal hygiene.

I don't call writing stuff down "journaling" because that's a big turnoff for lots of folks. I just call it "keeping a list." Every day, ever since COVID began, I write down whatever self-care practices I do that day to boost my personal well-being. I'm on book four, titled "The Things Are Getting Better" edition.

I'll jot down a morning yoga class, an after-work meditation, or a neighborhood bike ride with Abraham in the basket. A good cry counts. So does an ice-cold vodka martini, extra olives, with friends, outside, at whatever distance feels comfortable.

Of course, my entries vary daily. Many days, I take a walk. The days I mingle with the outside world, I come home and do the neti pot or hang my head over a pot of steaming water. In my house, that's what self-care looks like.

What I don't ever do is beat myself up if I have a lazy day or forget to make an entry. That can happen. That *does* happen. So, what? So, nothing. I'm an imperfect being doing the best I can. If I miss a day of keeping track—wait! what happened to Wednesday?—I laugh at myself and begin again.

Writing stuff down—yes, keeping a journal—is still one of the most powerful ways I know to stay on track with whatever you want for yourself in the future.

Adapt and survive. If I ever get a tattoo, that could be it.

3. I learned personal well-being is not a red-state-blue-state issue. It's about the state of your personal health, physical, mental, emotional, spiritual. Who among us—red state, blue state, even in our current state of COVID confusion and despair—isn't sick and tired of being sick and tired?

After the first edition of *All Is Well* came out, and before COVID-19 locked us down, I was able to travel freely around the country, talking to old people, young people, people of color, people of privilege, Republicans, Democrats, independents, libertarians, dog lovers, cat lovers, gun lovers…

We're all so different in so many ways, yes. But we're connected and united when it comes to one essential truth: Deep down, where our cells live and our molecules quiver, we aspire to be healthier, happier, less stressed, and more calm. The human body wants to be in balance, in homeostasis. More often than not, we get in our own way.

Living through COVID-19 taught me something I've learned before and I hope you have, too: We are one people, one human race, and to adapt and survive is in our DNA.

So, why did COVID kill more Americans than any other nationality on earth (as of this printing)? How did the politics of health care undermine the promise of health care?

I knew I'd want to touch on those prickly issues in a second edition. And I also knew I wanted to go through the first edition and take out any snide or partisan political remarks I might have made.

The fact is that I'm a trained journalist from back in the day when journalists had training. In this second edition, I'm not taking the side of the Republicans or the Democrats. I'm taking *your* side, dear reader, to help you discover your own path to well-being. You'll decide what direction you want to go.

4. I learned there are angels in this world. They are posing as health care professionals, frontline workers, and essential others who treat the sick, teach our kids, deliver the groceries, work at food pantries, bury our dead, and otherwise serve to help us get through the most trying times we've ever known.

A big lesson of COVID—for so many of us—is you can't say thank you enough. The mind attaches to the negative, so it's up to us to shift to the positive and see the amazing acts of kindness and goodness and compassion that are happening all around us, all the time, in hospitals, in schools, in backyards, on front stoops, and in all the places that people gather. I learned that being grateful every day for the life you have is what personal well-being feels like.

5. I learned that certain health care policies make no sense. In fact, they're destructive.

Here's what I mean. As we moved through this time of COVID, the public health messaging got clearer and clearer: Wear a mask; stay home; wash your hands; social distance; get the vaccine. That's the path forward, our most trusted doctors are still telling us day after day, week after week, more than a year into the virus.

But you know what they're not telling us? They're not telling us about the value of self-care. They're not telling us that every person has an innate immune system, and the stronger yours is, the more resilient you are, the greater your chance of surviving the virus, and others on their way, and getting on with your life.

Why have doctors been so silent about that? Sure, it's hard for people to make behavioral change, but we also know that a health scare—a heart attack, a cancer diagnosis, a deadly virus—can be a great motivator when it comes to self-care. That's why I'm sad and disappointed so many public-facing health experts missed the opportunity to tell people other scientifically proven methods for boosting your own immune system. Why is that?

Get plenty of sleep. Move your body every day. Eat real food, in appropriate amounts. Reach out to loving family and friends. Recognize the stress in your life, and find enjoyable ways to release and relax.

Occasionally, rarely, a public health official might mention a tip or two for healthier living, but for sure, advice about boosting your own immune system played out in a very minor key.

Self-care was *never* an official part of the mainstream messaging from our public health officials. Nor did the CDC come up with a recommended at-home protocol for people with early symptoms. Vaccines were pushed exclusively, and at-home treatment was not given the attention it deserves.

Why is that? Eventually, I learned to stop asking.

6. I learned that self-care is not selfish. It's not for rich folks; it's open to all. It's a way of moving through the world so the grief and pain and overwhelming

uncertainty of COVID don't leave you feeling lost and afraid. Instead, you find strength, perspective, and even joy in the most unexpected places. That's how you know you're engaged with your personal well-being. Like throwing up, you know when it's happening.

It's the misery-making part of COVID that taught me this undeniable truth: If you don't take good care of yourself, no one else will.

No one is coming to rescue you. That's why self-care exists. The government won't save you. Your money can't save you. The medical authorities have their hands full, and they might want to save you, but instead they're forced to leave you out in an overcrowded hospital hallway, on a gurney, no loved ones allowed, waiting for someone to come along and give you a drug or put you on a breathing machine that may or may not help you live another day.

This book can help you live another day…especially this braver, bolder, deeper, darker second edition…but not without your full cooperation. Your personal well-being depends on the choices you and only you can make.

Let's call that your path. Everyone has one. You're on yours right now. —Marilynn

Introduction.

It was 1972, in Chicago, and my husband and I made a bold and crazy decision to take our ten-speed bicycles to France and ride through the gorgeous vineyards of Bordeaux and Burgundy. We had no idea what we were getting into.

I decided I'd better "get in shape"—whatever that means—so one day I walked over to the park across from our apartment and went for a run. Only a few blocks, just to see how it felt.

I'll tell you how it felt. It was a near-death experience. My lungs nearly exploded. My heart was in my throat, the size of a honeydew. My legs—in complete shock—grew roots. I stumbled home and collapsed on my bed. I was out of breath, out of condition, and out of excuses: How could so little physical exercise make me feel like such a big lump of nothing good?

I somehow survived, loved that first bike trip to France, and came home with a bottomless curiosity to know more about my body and how to keep all its moving parts juiced and happy.

I've always been fascinated by the miracle that is the human body, how it works and plays. I grew up saying I wanted to be a doctor but never took a single pre-med course. After getting a master's degree in journalism, my first job was in New York as a science writer for *Medical World News*. But at the time of my doomsday running experience, I had a dream job at the *Chicago Tribune*, reviewing movies, theater, and TV, and interviewing way too many Hollywood celebrities.

I was also writing feature stories on pretty much whatever interested me, which allowed me many trips to La-La Land in the '70s to research these new things called "holistic health" and "integrative medicine" and the "mind-body connection."

It was all happening in California. In Chicago, in 1976, yoga and yogurt were interchangeable terms, and most people considered the mind-body connection another name for the neck.

After a few years of deeper exploration, including a five-part series on Pyramid Power, I went to Mike Argirion, the features editor at the *Tribune*, and pitched him on a new kind of medical column.

The traditional doctor columns were all about pills and pimples, headaches and hemorrhoids, but I wanted to talk to readers about fitness, wellness, injury prevention, stress reduction, smart eating, deep breathing, and a bunch of other subjects that now fit under the expanding and sustainable umbrella of "a healthy lifestyle."

Back then, a healthy lifestyle wasn't even a concept. Fitness was just beginning to creep into the consciousness of the nation, right up there with CB radio and needlepoint. Jane Fonda was in leg warmers, going for the burn; Jim Fixx was inspiring a running revolution; farmers markets were just for selling fresh corn; and only tough guys belonged to gyms.

Argirion liked my idea. "Bring me some samples," he said, and immediately I reached out to Dr. David Bachman, team physician for the Chicago Bulls, a highly respected sports medicine doc. Smart, easygoing, open-minded.

"It's a column for people like me," I explained to him, "ordinary mortals who want to live healthier, happier lives and need some sound advice about being active and getting fit without damaging vital parts or giving up red wine."

David liked the idea, too, so we teamed up. I created and wrote the column, and David made sure we were giving out safe, sensible, up-to-date information. It started off in the

Tribune's "Outside" section in September 1976 as a weekly Q&A column, and I named it "Dr. Jock" (after Dr. Spock): "I'm a runner with knee pain. What do I do?" Or, "How can I lose ten pounds by Christmas?"

It was a hit in Chicago and soon after became a nationally syndicated column running in dozens of newspapers around the country. David and I did a book together, *Dear Dr. Jock: The People's Guide to Sports and Fitness* (published by E.P. Dutton), and after he moved his practice to the ski mountains of Colorado, I collaborated on the column with Dr. Mitchell Sheinkop, a competitive triathlete and another outstanding sports medicine expert in Chicago.

Meanwhile, I was becoming a sports medicine expert myself, journalistically speaking, going way beyond the 10,000 hours mark, researching for columns, interviewing doctors and scientists, reading books, taking courses, living the life, and giving lots of healthy lifestyle talks and workshops. In 1996, I became an ACE-certified personal trainer and then a certified Wellcoach many years later. And after forty years writing what's become America's longest-running fitness column, I've never stopped being curious about what it means to live a vibrant, exciting, healthy, and happy life. (My latest discovery is the stand-up desk.)

A lot of what I've learned is in this book: forty chapters with titles that sound like directives but are really just guidelines. If there's one thing I've learned for sure, it's you can't tell another person what to do.

Well, you can, but it doesn't work. It's not an effective way to help people change. And helping women and men and kids of all ages make positive, powerful changes in their lives is at the heart of *All Is Well: The Art {and Science} of Personal Well-Being.*

Link Mind and Body. Live a Big, Juicy Life. Be Your

Own Uncle Sam. Explore Endlessly. Think In Pictures. Mind Your Menus. Practice De-Aging. Live Long, Die Happy.

Some essays will resonate. Others may sound like California dreaming. All are intended to help you discover what *you* personally value when it comes to living your best life, because that's the only way lifelong change is going to happen.

It's up to you, dear reader. I can inform, inspire, educate, amuse, cajole, and otherwise cheer you on, but when push comes to shove—two excellent ways to burn one hundred calories—you're in charge of your own personal well-being. And that's good news because the more you take charge, study up, and stay vigilant, the greater success you'll experience.

As for my successes over the years, and my failures, I am nothing but grateful. I eventually left that dream job at the *Tribune* to create and produce a nationally syndicated TV series on sports, fitness, and adventure called "Energy Express." It ran in 120 cities, won two Emmys, and was honored for excellence by the Women's Sports Foundation and the National Association of Television Programming Executives. In the early 2000s, I decided to make "Energy Express" the name of the column, too.

I've done many other things in my work life, including running a successful TV production company and having two plays produced, with a third one in the wings. I've performed on camera as the co-host of two TV series, including *Stay Tuned*, similar to the *Siskel & Ebert* movie review show, but featuring two TV critics. I am the founding chair of a life-changing nonprofit called Girls in the Game, and I still work as an enthusiastic board member, helping girls get the healthy lifestyle training they need to become strong, powerful women. I was also the managing partner of a startup that staged the world's first internet auction of independent films, and I wrote and produced a documentary in1986 called *Adventure Travel in Israel.*

I'll stop now.

The one true red thread that runs through everything I've done and believe in lives on in my writing, my website, and now this book: Be active. Practice kindness. Eat real food. Live your best life. Be happy. Be grateful. Help others.

All is well.

—Marilynn Preston

Winter

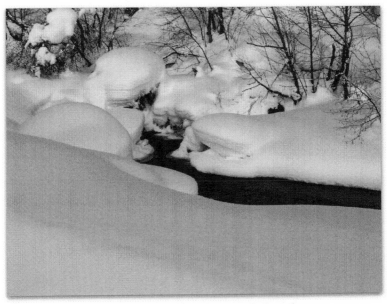

San Juan National Forest, Colorado

"I prefer winter and fall,
when you feel the bone structure of the landscape.
Something waits beneath it,
the whole story doesn't show."
—Andrew Wyeth

"Wintering is a metaphor for those phases in our life when we feel frozen out or unable to make the next step, and that can come at any time, in any season, in any weather; that it has nothing to do with the physical cold."
—Katherine May

"Winter spring summer or fall
All you have to do is call
And I'll be there
You've got a friend."
—Carole King

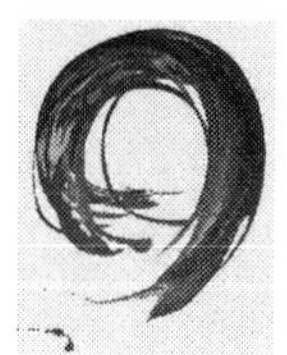

You always remember the First Time. And my first time experiencing the sensational connection between mind and body happened the weekend I turned thirty. It was an aikido workshop led by the late, great co-founder of the Human Potential Movement, George Leonard. "Make your arm strong!" he said. I stretched my right arm out and powered it up, squeezing as hard as I could until it was straight and strong. George pushed slightly and down it came, like a child poking at a balloon. Whoa! What just happened? George suggested a visualization. "Now release any tension, and imagine you're sending a beam of light through your arm, past your fingers, beyond the wall, down the street..." Strength through relaxation. I was a woman of steel. It was a mind-blowing, life-changing experience. If I can do this, I remember thinking, what else is possible?

Link Mind and Body.

I want to tell you three real-life stories to make one big point about the mind-body connection. It's real. It's not waiting to be proven someday; it *has* been proven, with scientific rigor, time and time again. Your mind and body are communicating with each other right now, inside you, hormonally, chemically, energetically, whether you're aware of it or not.

Becoming aware is a process of self-discovery and self-care, and it's never been more important than now, since the horrific and humbling global pandemic reshaped our world.

When you wake up to our new reality and sense the connections between your fears and emotions, and how your body might be expressing them—back pain, headaches, sleeplessness, indigestion, fatigue—it's a stunning aha! moment.

You won't blame yourself for every setback or sickness, but you'll become open to discovering that there are lessons to be learned, especially about the effects of stress on your health, healing, and well-being.

True story one: Sandy's husband died some months ago. They'd been together for nearly twenty-five years, a warm and compatible second marriage for both. Sandy depended on Bill, and Bill depended on Sandy, in a way that made them excited to be with each other, each trying to make the other happier.

Shortly after Bill died, Sandy stumbled and broke her foot. It was agony added to misery, and Sandy didn't understand why it happened.

"I know that Bill is watching over me…so why did I have to fall?"

In time, she answered her own question.

"I was moving too fast. I couldn't bear to be in the house without him, so I sold it right away and moved to a smaller place, and I've been making a lot of fast, reckless decisions ever since."

Sandy decided her broken foot was a sign to slow down, move more cautiously. It's not taking away her deep grief, Sandy says, but her mood is better, and she's making smarter decisions.

Story two: Lew is eighty-seven; his wife, Bonnie, is eighty-six, and they've been living happily, independently, outside Chicago, in a house they never want to leave. On a recent Sunday night, Bonnie was taken to the hospital because she had difficulty breathing. It was not a new problem, but it was a scary one. Lew spent the day with her in intensive care and came home to an empty house. He had some supper, put himself to bed, and woke up after a few hours, unable to move his legs. This had never happened before. Lew called a neighbor, who called 911, and after two days of hospital tests, his doctors could find nothing physical to explain his sudden paralysis.

"I didn't want to go on without her," Lew figured out the next day, after his legs returned to normal. "That's why my legs wouldn't work."

Lew is home now, and so is Bonnie, both grateful to be together again.

"The body is an amazing thing," Lew says. "It knows more than I do."

Story three: A married couple—tired of cold winters and in love with Northern California—went to look for a home in Marin County. They were all super expensive, so the couple decided they'd sell another piece of real estate they owned before buying something new in California.

But then the tireless realtor took them to see the house of their dreams.

"This is it!" they cheered, lost in real estate rapture. "We'll never find a better place!"

They bid on the house without waiting for the other property to sell, which involved a risky bridge loan, among other negatives. But what the heck, they high-fived: no guts, no glory.

The night before signing the offer, the wife suddenly felt the worst pain of her life gripping across her chest, lurching down her right arm. She hadn't fallen, lifted weights, or done a crooked handstand in yoga.

"Is this a heart attack?" she wondered. "No! It feels deeply muscular, like someone is twisting my arm."

Her partner jumped to the exact right conclusion.

"We're not buying the house! Look what your body is telling us. If you can't move your right arm, you can't sign the offer. Forget it. We'll wait until the time is right."

The next day, the wife saw a wise body worker, fluent in neuromuscular stress, and by noon, her arm was ninety-five percent better.

And she used it to hug her most understanding partner.

ENERGY EXPRESS-O! All Is One

"Body is not stiff, mind is stiff."
—K. Pattabhi Jois

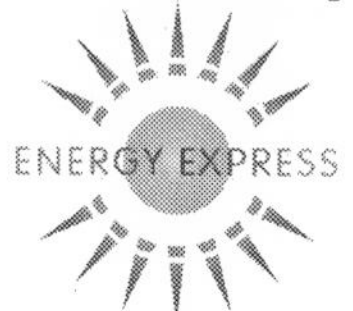

GOING DEEPER

If you can't describe *your* first time experiencing the mind-body connection, don't worry.

Just know it's not too late. Decide for yourself that you want to experience that sweet spot when mind and body are linked without struggle, and you feel calmer, clearer, more focused, less frightened.

There are many paths to this felt sense of well-being, but reading about it won't take you there. It's an experience, and it can't come from books. You need curiosity, an open mind, a teacher, a training, and, most of all, an actual practice that helps you plug into the electrifying flow of energy that develops when your body and mind work in harmony.

Yoga is famous for it. So is impeccable training in the martial arts, including Qigong, tai chi, and aikido. The Alexander Technique can take you there, and so can Feldenkrais, somatics training, and Pilates.

What about fishing? Yes! Hiking in a forest? Absolutely! Posting your twentieth tweet of the day? Not so much.

Once you have that felt sense of a body-mind connection, you'll want to keep coming back to that sweet spot time and again. Your practice never gets tiresome or boring. Instead, it becomes a way of seeing the clarity behind the chaos, the interconnectedness of *all* things, inner and outer, humans and rocks, the sea and the stars.

Start where you are. Even in the grip of COVID-19, even if you've never felt the connection before, it is there, waiting for you.

Some changes happen to you for no good reason, like the pandemic, like losing your job or your business or your darling one. Other changes happen because of you, the result of deep personal effort. How is it that some people can sober up or slim down or let go of crippling emotions like anger and guilt, while others stay stuck in the paralyzing groove of woulda, shoulda, coulda? I've trained to be a Wellcoach to get to the heart of that mystery. It's more about your readiness to change and less about a will of iron. Positive thinking is a lifesaver, no matter what kind of change you're facing. You need to believe you can always begin again.

Begin. Again.

I can't say the new year that began to unfold in early January 2021 was even close to normal. We were locked up, shut down, and experiencing the most frightening health scare in one hundred years.

And still, we felt that perfectly normal urge to make New Year's resolutions, most having to do with living a happier, healthier, less stressful, and more satisfying life. Red state, blue state, we all want to experience that unifying state of well-being, don't we?

"I want to start exercising every day!"

"I'm going to sit still and do nothing for ten minutes every morning."

"I want to play more, work less…learn to cook…cut out diet sodas…restore my '67 Mustang…give up being perfect…untether from devices during meals…"

It's your call, your choice, your personal vision of what your best self looks like in the year ahead. The work is to create the vision—for yourself, your family, your company—and strive toward it, step by step, sometimes taking a step back but always looking forward.

And here's the essential question: If you dream it, can you do it? The answer that serves you best is yes. Like plants turning to the light, we humans are capable of turning our lives around and making smarter choices.

As your most personal trainer, I must tell you that the odds are against you. Statistically, backsliding is to behavior change as slicing is to golf. The mind attaches to the negative. Remember that the next time you beat yourself up for skipping a workout. Your mind doesn't like change, actually resists it, and it will invent clever ways to throw you off course. Experts tell us that most people will fail to keep their New Year's resolutions within the first three months.

But here's the good news: You are not most people. You are uniquely you, hard-wired and biochemically organized to change your life in profound ways if and when you are motivated and ready. Neuroscience tells us the brain is capable of rewiring, but it's up to us to play chief electrician.

In other words, genuine and long-lasting lifestyle change is possible. Take it from someone who had a near-death experience at thirty when she tried to run a mile. You must trust in yourself—really! truly! deeply!—because the more you believe you *can* do something, the more likely you *will* do it.

That relationship between belief and action is called self-efficacy, a key concept that enables you to defy the odds and make New Year's resolutions that last, if not a lifetime, at least several nourishing years. And then, as always, you can begin again.

To make change happen in your life, it helps to understand how change happens. For that, please turn to more than twenty-five years of research by Dr. James Prochaska and colleagues, authors of the classic book *Changing for Good*, an excellent guide to help you move from not thinking about change to thinking about it, to planning for it, to doing it, to maintaining the change for a lifetime.

One of Prochaska's pearls (or is it a thorn?) is that if you're not ready for change, it won't happen. Don't beat yourself up or waste your time. But when you are ready, it can happen. Obstacles are overcome, and single-minded determination kicks in. How do you know if you're ready? Keep reading.

Go inside. You can't calm your mind, lose weight, and commit yourself to daily movement routines just because your spouse, doctor, or insurance company wants you to. You need to dig deep and decide for yourself: Am I truly ready to change? Am I done with the excuses, the drama, the need to feel shame and blame? What are the pros? What are the cons? Write it down. Think it through. If you need coaching help, get it.

When the pros of making change outweigh your cons, you're ready for the next step: identifying the challenges involved and coming up with specific strategies to overcome them. You can't rush through or fake this self-discovery phase. Well, you can...but your lifestyle change will last as long as a bad pedicure.

Set realistic goals. Unrealistic goals—"I'll lose twenty pounds by Valentine's Day!"—set you up for failure. Can you starve, deny, torture yourself? Sure. But it's dumb and teaches you nothing about healthy eating. If you remember nothing else about goal setting, remember this: You want to be successful.

Scale down your goals to bite-sized, doable challenges—a one-minute meditation practice, a meatless Monday, two thirty-minute walks a week instead of four. The point is to feel successful on a weekly basis. Small victories boost your confidence and motivate you to stay on track.

Be specific, or nothing will change. Don't vaguely tell yourself to cut out sweets, for instance. Decide on the details: Snack on seven almonds instead of a handful of M&M's, or switch your morning muffin for a bowl of unsweetened yogurt, walnuts, and some blueberries.

If it's physical fun, aka exercise, you want more of, be specific about what you'll do and when. Schedule workouts on your calendar. "Speed-walk for thirty minutes around the neighborhood on Tuesday morning, starting at 7 a.m." Details make all the difference!

Slow down, and be patient. Change is not linear. It's often two steps forward, one stumble back. Some days, the best part of your workout is simply showing up. Accept that. New habits take the time they take. It might happen suddenly—or it might not. Make your best effort; let go of the result; and stick with it.

The positive change you want for yourself—like eating meals made of real food, for example—could take months to become a comfortable part of your life. So what? The bigger the hurry, the smaller the reward.

When you feel yourself slipping and falling—and you will!—get back up, and begin again. That's what resilience feels like. Plan for success. And if you're fooling yourself and unwilling to do the work of change, accept it. For now.

As my favorite Jedi master and wellness coach, Yoda, revealed years ago:

"Do. Or do not. There is no try."

When you're ready to change, you don't try. You do.

ENERGY EXPRESS-O! Ready, Set, Go

"People don't resist change. They resist being changed."
—Peter Senge

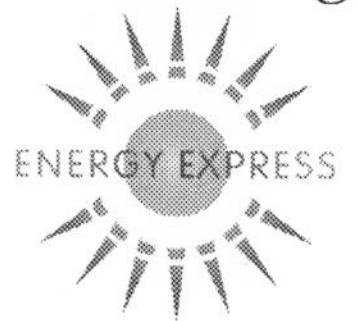

GOING DEEPER

One day, maybe when it's cold and drizzling outside, decide to create a wellness vision for yourself. No experience necessary.

Lots of people ended up doing some form of this during COVID-19. They had time; they had anxiety; they knew they weren't living their best life.

As a result, overworked adults discovered the simple joys of family dinners, and city folk moved to the country to raise goats, and people learned how good it felt to bake your own bread, deepen your relationships, learn to play chess.

Wellness visions can lead you where you want to go, if you really focus on the life you want to live.

Be brave.

To get started, sit comfortably, inhale, and exhale slowly and gently, in and out of your nose; imagine yourself a year from now, living a life that is happier, healthier, and more fulfilling, whatever that means to you.

Paint the picture in glorious detail. What, specifically, are you doing? How are you feeling? Are you alone or with other people? Name their names. See their faces. Feel your joy.

Enjoy the process, and when you're finished detailing your wellness vision, write it down and read it back to yourself, out loud. People believe what they hear themselves say, any good wellness coach will tell you. So say it loud; say it proud; and don't get tangled up in judgment. It's your vision, your life, and it will be up to you to make it happen.

Here's an example to inspire you, taken from the wellness vision of a frustrated but determined woman I worked with who went on to make remarkable changes in her own life.

"I see myself playing with my grandchildren at the beach, and my back pain is gone, and I'm not ashamed of how I look in a swimsuit because I'm having a fabulous time, and I feel loved and liberated."

Once you're satisfied with your wellness vision, you'll want a detailed plan to make it happen. If you can team up with a gifted coach or community counselor, please do. An empathic friend with good listening skills can also help. You'll have to lead the way, but you'll have a partner to dance with, an ally who helps you resolve your ambivalence and build on your strengths.

We don't change because some healthy lifestyle expert comes along and tells us we should. We change when we are ready. Having a wellness vision can help us get ready.

And besides all that, it's just a fun thing to do on a rainy afternoon.

Why is it so hard to slow down and savor the moment? Because the mind is like a monkey, the Buddhists tell us, and neuroscientists agree, always jumping from one thing to the next, from the past to the future and back again, often negative, the opposite of steady and calm. Getting through the COVID crisis has been universally exhausting and depleting, and it's also been revealing. Most of us are more connected to our computers than we are to our calm center. But this is our modern world. We are online, on call, on Zoom, on edge, and under surveillance many hours every day. What can we do?

Slo-o-o-ow Down.

Are you in a big hurry to slow down?

I am. Moving slowly is the secret to a life well lived, a Zen master once told me, but it took COVID-19 to convince me.

For millions, our experience of time shifted, and so did our priorities. Nowhere to go, everything to do, including finding a calm and safe center to ride out the uncertainty, the grief, the hidden blessings.

For this, we do yoga. There are other paths to personal well-being, but this one is so available, with an estimated 300 million practitioners around the planet. As you've guessed, I'm one of them.

Yoga can give you an inner awareness of slowing down, if you've got a skilled teacher giving you the right cues, not speeding you up so you jump mindlessly from pose to pose. That's when injuries happen—and oh, boy, do they! By slowing down, not only are you unlikely to hurt yourself, but you also open up to the transformative magic that happens when you move frame by frame, breath by breath.

I had some profound peeks into that magic some time ago, when about fifty-eight of us put our mats down in a huge tent at Esalen, the renowned retreat center devoted to exploring human potential, perched on the spectacular coastline in Big Sur, California. We were there to dive deeply into the Zen of Slowing Down, a five-day workshop led by Tias Little and Henry Shukman.

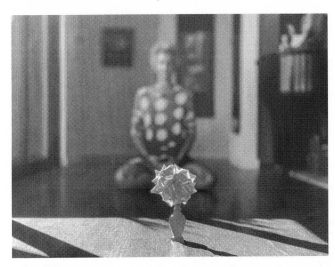

Tias is a master yoga teacher, and Henry is a master Zen teacher. They are also writers, poets, philosophers, and good friends and students of each other, as well as friends of mine. Their yoga and Zen centers in Santa Fe, New Mexico, are only a mile and a half apart. What a coincidence.

"In an age of acceleration, nothing can be more exhilarating than going slow," Henry reads to us at the start of the week, quoting Pico Iyer.

"In an age of constant distraction, nothing is so luxurious as paying attention.

"In an age of constant movement, nothing is so urgent as sitting still."

Sitting still. Paying attention. Going slow. All that, plus Esalen's soothing tubs, wild waves, passing dolphins, and exquisite home-grown vegetables served up at community dinners that have the look, feel, and feathers of a Federico Fellini film.

I want to share a few highlights of the workshop because

Tias and Henry have many wise teachings to offer. But first, I promise you that you don't have to go to Esalen or a hermit's cave to begin to slow down your own busy life.

As Henry says—a core truth at the heart of many teachings—"Start where you are." Accepting yourself and your life just as they are allows for change to happen, and from that place, you can begin to let go of an accelerated pace of life that makes your hamstrings tight, your low back sore, your heart constricted.

Paying attention—being in the moment—is a crucial part of slowing down. It can happen anywhere, anytime. For many people, being forced to slow down, way down, was one of the unexpected silver linings of the COVID-19 crisis. Once you taste it, it's hard to forget.

Back to Esalen. When we did walking meditation outside with Henry, we got into the groove of being in the moment by paying strict attention to the soles of our feet. It's not easy. The mind is like a monkey...but breathing it back into the soles of our feet is what the mind-body connection feels like.

When you do yoga with Tias Little, the focus is not only on the alignment of the pose but also—always!—on how it *feels*. Inside. The vibrations, the pulsations, the sensations of prana—our life force—that flow through us and light the body electric.

The deep somatic work Tias guides us through at the start of class is called SATYA, Tias's name for Sensory Awareness Training for Yoga Attunement.

It's done on our backs, on our blankets, and requires us to direct our awareness to what's going on inside and around our spines, our lungs, our shoulder blades, our selves.

It looks like we're doing nothing when, in fact, we're doing some of the most profound and subtle work you can do to prevent injuries and increase your strength. We are sensing; we are feeling; we are using our mind's eye to direct energy and insight to the only body we get in this lifetime.

Are my kidneys floating? Is my sacrum level? Can I squeeze muscle to bone and draw energy up the inside of my legs? Is my heart open? Are the four corners of my feet pressing down into the floor, into the earth?

If you stop to let your rational mind question, then you've lost the moment of influencing the subtle body, the theme of a recent Tias book, *Yoga of the Subtle Body*.

Tias's style of mind-body training—very precise, very playful—enables his students to develop our somatic intelligence.

And that—along with a lot of time spreading my sitting bones—has guided me to an understanding of what a profound, self-healing practice yoga can be.

"The everyday world we live in values accomplishment, achieving, acquiring," Henry says, as we all nod and know the truth of that and the stress of that.

We are all scrambling to have the best house, the best job, the best car. "What if we let ourselves be as we are?" Henry asks. "Why hurry up? Why not enjoy the ride?"

Your body is alive with pulsating rhythms as energy flows in your cells, brain, joints, muscles, and tissues. Tias tells us that if we can slow down enough to tune in—through sensing, breathing, and meditation—we can help the body heal, stay healthy, and even glow.

"It's like a light shining from within," he quotes Ged Sumner and Steve Haines. "It's the glow of life that can be seen in the skin, eyes, and the aura."

Fear not, dear reader! You don't have to believe in your aura to go for the glow. It's what vibrant health looks like. You might see it in the mirror one day, and slowing down is one deeply satisfying way to make it happen.

For more on the transformative ways of Tias and Henry, check out their websites, prajnayoga.com and mountaincloud.org.

As for Esalen, it's one of the best places on earth to learn to open your heart, soothe your brain, and float your kidneys.

ENERGY EXPRESS-O! Other Worldly

"I have lived with several Zen masters—all of them cats."
—Eckhart Tolle

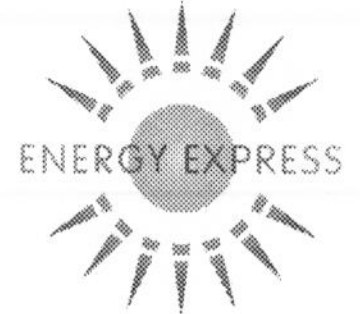

GOING DEEPER

Are you willing to try a walking meditation? It's a taste of what slowing down feels like.

Here's a summary of Henry's step-by-step teaching:

Step 1: Walk in nature. Sometimes, walking meditation is done inside a Zen temple—a break from long periods of sitting meditation—but doing it outside, in nature, offers special benefits. Wear comfortable shoes and appropriate clothes, and pick a path that is safe and unencumbered.

Step 2: Arrange your hands. There is a Zen way of doing just about everything—from eating a meal to being with your dog—so it's no surprise that walking meditation in Henry's Sanbo-Zen lineage has rules about how to hold your hands.

"You put your right hand around your right thumb and

use the left hand to gently press your right hand against your solar plexus, just below the diaphragm, the energetic center of strength, confidence, and joy," Henry demonstrated. "That's the Zen way."

Is it the only way? Of course not. It's so not Zen to dictate to people what they can and can't do.

Step 3: Mind your posture. Walking meditation needn't be reminiscent of a funeral march. Follow the rules, but also follow your bliss. Walk mindfully, in silence, with an upright spine and a slight chin tuck. Your eyes are open and lowered, but not in a way that makes your walking unsafe. Personally, I like to throw in a serene smile.

Walk in a way that feels relaxed and aware, opening up the deepest channels of the body, allowing for a flow of energy up and down the spine, drawing up from the earth, drawing down from the sky. I know it sounds a little woo-woo, but so what? Lots of things that used to seem woo-woo are now known to be true-true.

Step 4: Don't focus on your breath. Really? "Let your mind rest in the soles of your feet," Henry told us. Don't overthink it. Just let go, and let it happen, walking at a comfortable pace, focusing your mind's eye on the bottom of your feet.

When you lose focus—and you will, just like in sitting meditation—you simply acknowledge the lapse, congratulate yourself for noticing, return your awareness to the soles of your feet, and keep it there until your walk is finished.

Step 5: Nothing to gain. At the end of our refreshing and revelatory twenty-minute walking meditation, Henry explained a little more about its power.

"It's about being as we are, where we are…the experience of the now. Our minds grasp for meaning, grasp for understanding…

"There is nothing to understand," said Henry, "There is just now."

This chapter—"Be a Mouth Taper"—is new to the second edition, all about the extraordinary healing power of nasal breathing. If there were ever a secret weapon, a natural quick-fix that protects your health and helps prevent physical and mental illness, nasal breathing is it. Hard to believe? Yes! So, please, lean in. Nasal breathing is what links your mind to your body in a way that calms your nervous system, helps you sleep, boosts your energy, and so much more. The mouth is for eating; the nose is for breathing—slow, conscious inhales and exhales in and out of your nose, not your mouth, as often as you can, during the day and all through the night. That's where the mouth taping comes in. The first time I tried it, I thought I'd wake up dead. But no. My breathing teachers were right: I woke up feeling rested, at ease, grateful. Some dear friends are intrigued. Others think I'm obsessed with this nasal breathing thing, and they're right; I am. During COVID, especially, it's been a lifesaver and a game changer, helping me stay healthy, strong, and wildly curious why our doctors don't recommend it. "I'd get too much pushback," a well-respected pulmonologist told me, in confidence. Yes, breathing exercises work, and no, they're not routinely discussed with patients who would benefit. When that changes, we can all breathe easier. After a year of study and research, and many months of a breathing practice that includes mouth taping, I've come to love sealing my lips with a small piece of paper tape every night. You know that feeling when your feet are cold in bed and you slip on a pair of warm socks just before closing your eyes? It feels like that. All is well.

Be a Mouth Taper.

Why learn to breathe through your nose? What's wrong with mouth breathing, which about ninety percent of us do, all day and night? It seems to be working, right? People aren't keeling over in the streets because they breathe in and out of their mouths thousands of times a day, right?

Yes and no. Nasal breathing is much, *much* healthier for

you than mouth breathing, and I intend to touch on why that is in this chapter. But I'm not going to spend all my time explaining the science behind nasal breathing because journalist James Nestor did that brilliantly in his 2020 bestseller, *Breath: The New Science of a Lost Art.*

If you haven't read it, please do. I've gifted at least fifteen friends and family members with a copy. I'm thrilled he wrote it so I don't have to.

"There is nothing more essential to our health and well-being than breathing: take air in, let it out, repeat 25,000 times a day," you'll read in *Breath*. "Yet, as a species, humans have lost the ability to breathe correctly, with grave consequences."

Grave consequences! That's what I was trying to avoid at the beginning of COVID because I'd had wicked bad pneumonia a few months before, and I'm considered old, and my lungs were vulnerable. I was scared.

All the advice I was hearing made sense—wash your hands; wear a mask; social distance; stay home—but I wasn't hearing anything from our trusted medical authorities about what I could do to make my lungs healthier, happier, less likely to succumb.

And then I started reading books, taking workshops, and learning about the protective power of nasal breathing. It wasn't just a lightbulb going off; it was a house full of lightbulbs, an exploding galaxy of lightness and brightness that revealed a whole world of modern research, ancient teachings, and cutting-edge studies in human physiology, biochemistry, and pulmonology that I wasn't aware of before.

And if I didn't know much about the benefits of nasal breathing—after forty-three years of writing America's longest-running fitness column—how could I expect my dear readers to know? I knew about pranayama, and I could comfortably breathe in and out of my nose during a vigorous ninety-minute yoga class, but I never thought about taking my breathing practice off the mat. Duh.

"Breathing, as it happens, is more than just a biochemical or physical act," Nestor writes. "It's more than just moving the diaphragm downward and sucking in air to feed hungry cells and remove wastes.

"The tens of billions of molecules we bring into our bodies with every breath also serve a more subtle, but equally important role. They influence nearly every internal organ, telling them when to turn on and off. They affect heart rate, digestion, moods, attitudes; when we feel aroused, and when we feel nauseated. Breathing is a power switch to a vast network called the autonomic nervous system."

And so much more. So, let me give you a few more of my most important discoveries after taking such a deep dive into nasal breathing, starting with amazing things I learned in a six-week, online, intensive class called Breath as Medicine, led by a very intense and skilled breathing master named Ed Harrold, author of *Life With Breath.*

1. Nasal breathing helps us cope with extreme challenges.

"We're living in extremely challenging times," breathing coach and educator Ed Harrold told us in my first Zoom session of his Breath as Medicine course, just as COVID was spreading terror and trauma throughout the world. "Let's do some breathing so we can get grounded in our body, heart, and brain so we can be as mindful as possible about the choices in our lives."

Mouth breathing won't do that, Ed knows. That's why he teaches athletes, business leaders, and anyone who's interested in the science behind nasal breathing—slow, deep, focused, using your diaphragm, hearing yourself make the sound of the ocean.

These conscious breathing techniques are self-care tools, Ed says, "designed to restore and repair your biochemical, biomechanical, physiological, and psychological health and well-being."

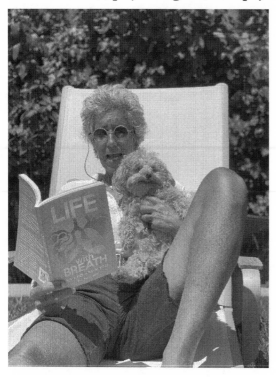

That translates into lowering your heart rate and blood pressure, reducing inflammation and oxidative stress, strengthening the immune system, stimulating the flow of nitric oxide, slowing the aging process, burning fat…and the list of proven benefits goes on.

After six weeks with Ed, not only could I imagine my brain rewiring—as he promised it would—but I also had a much better handle on my fear and anxiety. And that's because another one of the benefits of nasal breathing is that it engages the parasympathetic nervous system, and that calms us down and tells the brain we're safe and it can relax.

Let your own brain ease back to basic biology. Your autonomic nervous system has two co-equal branches. Your sympathetic nervous system is all about fight or flight or freeze, and the parasympathetic is rest and digest, relax and restore.

Both systems are crucial to your well-being and have to be in balance, and that's why nasal breathing is such a gift: It engages your parasympathetic system, giving you a level of clarity and inner calm that lets you perform at your highest level, whether you're a professional runner or a stay-at-home dad.

"We can be the smartest person in the world," says Ed, experienced, enthusiastic, fluent in mindfulness-based strategies, "but without the emotional intelligence that comes from being calm, centered and present, we'll be swimming upstream our entire lives."

2. Nasal breathing boosts your nitric oxide.

In 1998, three U.S. scientists won the Nobel Prize for discovering how important nitric oxide is in the human body. NO is called the "miracle molecule," a potent neurotransmitter that dilates and cleans lung tissue, helps lower blood pressure, aids the immune system, and decreases the likelihood of blood clots.

Another part of the miracle is that nitric oxide is produced inside the nasal cavity and transferred to the lower airways and lungs through nasal breathing. Nasal breathing, NOT mouth breathing.

"If we breathe through the mouth, we are missing the enormous benefit of nitric oxide, as it's not produced in the mouth," explains Sienna Smith, one of my favorite yoga and breathing teachers before, during, and after COVID.

Sienna's teachings are precise, passionate, and immensely helpful. I started off Zooming one of her five-day Breathing Boot Camps and continued along with her many morning workshops. Eventually, I did a remarkable twenty-one-day Breathe Well challenge that really got my own practice going, imperfect as it is.

"The first step to working with the breath is getting out of our way," Sienna teaches. Before you learn the many different techniques for controlling your breath—alternate nostril breathing, power breathing, breath holding—Sienna wants you to begin just noticing your natural breath.

"Natural breath is about allowing the breath to be as it appears now," she says. "Notice the quality of the breath. Without judging or assessment, notice the texture, pace, flow rate, and overall quality of the natural breath. It's like watching a play, and the main actor on stage is our breath. Witness the breath with curiosity, openness, and kindness."

3. Your lungs have no muscles.

Did you know your lungs have no muscles of their own? Of course not. Why do you need to? You're breathing now, and when you stop breathing, you're dead. In between, you go for checkups and hope nothing bad happens.

Here's the thing: Your lungs are made of tissue, and your lungs work much better when that tissue is dilated, clean, and energized. Breathing in and out inflates and deflates your lungs, and so does movement—expanding your chest; lifting your arms above your head and lowering them below your waist; moving your spine and torso up and down, front and back, side to side.

Lungs love that stuff. Those little squeezes and pumping actions make the juices flow so the lung tissue is nourished and there's less inflammation and more space for the proper exchange of oxygen in, carbon dioxide out.

In other words, Inhalators R Us. But when we lead sedentary lives, breathe in toxic air, and only breathe through our mouths, our lungs become compromised. We get lung cancer, asthma, and chronic obstructive pulmonary disease (COPD)—and, yes, some of us get COVID. Is nasal breathing a guarantee you won't get sick? No. Nothing is, not even the vaccines. But it's a powerful self-help tool.

4. Nasal breathing works.

I know what you're thinking. If nasal breathing works so well to improve your health and well-being, why isn't it right up there with masks, vaccines, and hand-washing in terms of recommended things to do to lower your risk of getting the coronavirus?

Great question! If I ever discover the answer, I may have to write a third edition. Meanwhile, let me tell you a story about a time it worked wonders for me. This is what's known as anecdotal evidence, something I absolutely believe in, as most people do.

In March 2021, I had to go to my doctor for a pre-op exam to get ready for a cataract operation. Usually, I don't have my doctor take my blood pressure because I believe in White Coat Syndrome and my numbers can come in a little too high. I'm not worried about hypertension, and neither is my doctor, but this time, she had to take it because the form she was filling out called for it.

"Okay," I said. "Take it."

The top number was 168, not good but not horrible.

"Fine," I said. "Just use that."

My doctor wrote it down, but she also said something smart, which is why she's my doctor.

"In a few minutes, you're going to take an EKG," Sally said. "Why don't you see if you can get that number down."

Sally knows about my obsession with nasal breathing. I smiled, but she was serious.

It was my first EKG ever, and attaching all those leads to my chest did nothing to calm me down. But still, I closed my eyes, found my diaphragm, and began to lower it and lift it, breathing slowly and deeply in and out of my nose.

It didn't feel relaxing. I was nervous. My breath was

raggedy, not smooth, and extending my exhale felt forced instead of fluid.

I did it anyway, and after a few minutes, the nurse took my blood pressure. The top number was 120. That's a 48-point improvement after a few minutes of focused nasal breathing. The lower number was better, too.

The nurse looked at me, looked at the number Sally had recorded, and said she needed to take it again. The second time, it was also 120. The EKG went well, too.

"Every breath we take tells our brain something about our emotional state," Harrold writes in *Life With Breath*. "When our hearts beat fast, our brain senses danger, and this perpetuates the chronic state of fight-or-flight that many people experience when there's no real threat of danger.

"On the other hand, when we breathe slowly, we lower our heart rate, and that tells our brain to relax, expand awareness, and learn new things."

I'm learning new things about the breath every day. You can learn, too, if you decide to. And if you stick with it, you'll be as astonished by the results as I am.

And for that, I am eternally, and internally, grateful.

ENERGY EXPRESS-O! Now You Know Everything

"The secret to health, fitness, and weight loss lies in how you breathe."

—Patrick McKeown

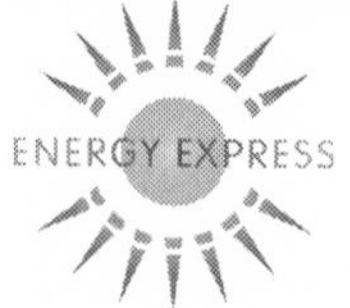

GOING DEEPER

To go deeper into nasal breathing, you need to experience it for yourself. Read books; take classes; and slowly, gradually, build up your own practice. It may not come quickly. That's fine. It takes the time it takes. You can't rush slowing down.

Books: Here are five terrific resources, starting with one by Tias Little, who brings powerful imagery, poetry, and wisdom to his understanding of the breath, the body, and the path:

The Practice is the Path by Tias Little (prajnayoga.com)

The Oxygen Advantage: Simple, Scientifically Proven Breathing Techniques To Help You Become Healthier, Slimmer, Faster, and Fitter by Patrick McKeown (oxygenadvantage.com and buteykoclinic.com)

Breath: The New Science of a Lost Art by James Nestor (mrjamesnestor.com)

Life With Breath by Ed Harrold (edharrold.com)

Pranayama Beyond the Fundamentals by Richard Rosen (richardrosenyoga.com)

Breathing teachers: You can easily find Ed Harrold and Patrick McKeown videos all over the internet. They detail how and why nasal breathing works, and they also teach specific exercises designed to help you with everything from asthma to Zoom fatigue.

Nathan James is another breathing teacher I respect and recommend. He coaches on Zoom, and you can reach him at www.therapeuticbodyworkcenter.com. It was Nathan who first told me I was an overbreathing mouth breather—really? me? fast and shallow?—and from there, all good things happened.

Sienna Smith has been an invaluable guide to life-saving breathing practices since COVID began. You can find her many online offerings—yoga, breathing, anatomy, and transformative therapeutic classes—at SiennaSmith.com. Sienna is also venturing out with her own podcast, *Breathe Better*, widely available.

"Ultimately," says Sienna, "a nasal breath that is even, moderately deep, effortless, soft, and slow is the most healthy way to breathe on all levels."

Even if I never get there, I'm happy to know I'll die trying.

Many people hibernate in winter. I can't bear the thought. I grew up on the South Side of Chicago (in what is now called Michelle Obama's neighborhood), and I used to hate the cold. Brrr-rrr-rr-r stands for brutal, blaming Mother Nature for my suffering. Hunched shoulders, frozen frown, bad attitude. But once I began to accept winter, my resistance melted, and the cold play of pleasure seeped into every cell. Learning to layer helped a lot. So did learning to ski. And when I discovered snowshoeing, I was in a state of bliss. So, this winter, put on a wild furry hat and find the winter sport that calls to you, or at least doesn't kill you.

Go Play in the Snow.

My friend's son broke several moving parts in a preventable snowboarding accident. It was serious. He'll spend months in rehab, and his stressed-out parents will spend thousands in medical fees.

Jake's a smart kid, a sophomore in college, athletic and strong. It turns out he was a big fan of the Winter Olympics and spent hours watching all those champion snowboarders do their somersaults, twists, and 360 big spins.

Awesome! Cool!

When Jake had his chance to go snowboarding, he pretty much lost his mind. Maybe his helmet was too tight. He decided to try a simple kickflip. No big deal, he thought. It's a beginner trick. He'd seen it done hundreds of times.

Of course, it was an insane move on his part. No training. No coaching. Just Jake and his brand-new Burton sliding down a mountain in Colorado, young and fearless and hoping for the best.

The best thing that happened is that he lived.

The flip side of Jake's story involves Janet, a woman I met recently at a fundraiser for old-growth forests. She, too, was inspired by the Winter Olympics. After a few nights of watching the skaters, she decided to go back to figure skating—after a fifty-year hiatus. She loved skating when she was a kid but gave it up to live her grown-up life, enjoy her family, and, over time, gain about thirty-five pounds.

"I was watching Kim Yuna…and all of a sudden, something inside of me called out." she told me. "I can do that! I used to do that! I want to do it again!" She felt a shift, and she acted on it.

Janet's joined a skating club and has taken eight lessons. She's sleeping better, feeling perkier, and—oh, yes—she's gone from a size 14 to a size 12 without even trying.

Have you found your cold-weather sport yet? If yes, what are you doing this winter to get better at it? Learning new things builds your brain and your confidence.

If you don't have a winter sport, what are you waiting for? (Nope, the answer isn't "summer.") Get outside; get moving; see what all the excitement's about. Hibernation—so good for bears, so not good for humans—tends to layer on the pounds and depress the spirit.

How to find your winter sport. This is our interactive moment. Let your mind play with the question: What winter sport calls to you? Snowshoeing? Cross-country skiing? Don't be ashamed to say curling.

Once you have your answer, make your move. Take a lesson. Join a club. Listen to that inner voice. It's the healthiest part of you, longing to breathe hard and feel the exhilaration and joy of being outdoors in the snow and ice, having your best time. And it's so *beautiful* out there.

Learn to layer. Dressing for cold-weather workouts is simple once you understand the basics of layering. The garment closest to your skin should be a performance fabric that wicks away your moisture, your sweat. That means give up your cottons. When cotton gets wet, it stays wet, and that can make you feel cold and uncomfortable when the temperature drops. The top layer depends on how active you will be. Many downhill skiers favor down. A cross-country skier would faint in a heavy down jacket. Just make sure your top-layer jacket is waterproof and wind-resistant.

Cross-country versus downhill. Skiing is a magnificent sport in all its forms, but there are big differences between cross-country and downhill. Cross-country is aerobic and will boost your fitness. Do it long enough and often enough, and it will get you into the shape of your life. That's not true of downhill skiing, which is really a controlled fall. To ski well and safely, you need to develop strength and flexibility off the slopes.

Downhill also costs a lot more than cross-country. Both sports offer plenty of thrills, chills, and magic. Whichever you choose, prepare with sport-specific training to develop balance and flexibility; take lessons; and bring your mind into play.

If you're still turning a cold shoulder to being outdoors in winter—throwing another log on the fire as you read this—accept that, and keep moving…indoors.

You can choose from a zillion Zoom workouts—another perk of the pandemic—or you can save up and buy one piece of sturdy home-fitness gear: a stationary bike, a rower, an elliptical cross trainer. It's your choice.

That'll keep you in a stay-at-home sweat till you see your first robin, or till we get the "COVID All-Clear" sign, whenever and however that happens.

ENERGY EXPRESS-O! Laugh at the Cold

"The problem with winter sports is that—follow me closely here—they generally take place in winter."
—Dave Barry

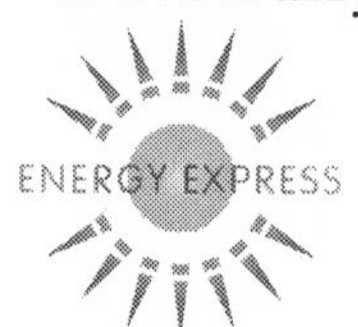

GOING DEEPER

COVID put outdoor activity into a deep freeze for a while, but we know it's coming back.

So stay chill, and try this: Plan a day of winter-sport wackiness with family and friends. Try to find a physical activity no one's done before.

What would be pure fun? Sledding? Ice fishing? Snow-person building?

I'll never forget playing my one and only round of Goofy Golf in the North Woods of Wisconsin. I was dressed in multicolored down from head to toe. It was way below zero, and there was three feet of snow on the ground.

We stood on an old used tire, teed up a bright yellow golf ball, and swung away into the frozen wilderness with vintage clubs that hadn't seen the inside of a golf bag in decades. What a hoot!

And yes, it involved a bar.

Call me crazy, but I've always been very protective of my brain. Without it, I'd be nothing. I follow neuroscience the way some people follow the Chicago Cubs, and along the way, I've learned my brain is happiest when it's rested, nurtured, and organized—AND challenged, stimulated, and well-fed. All of that has made me wary of too much time with technology. I'm not anti-anything, pretty much, but I'm super cautious about filling my brain with input from my digital devices. Is technology moving us forward in our thinking, or is it pulling us away from the kind of quiet reflective time the brain needs to make sense of our world and our best place in it? The pace of life is so much quicker, while destructive plaque grows so much thicker, so it's up to us to practice self-care and keep our precious brains juiced and jubilant for as long as we can.

Grow Your Gray Matter.

It wasn't long ago that our best and brightest doctors thought the brain had a built-in "stop" button and it naturally ceased growing and gradually shut down as we got older. Bummer.

Also completely untrue. (Doesn't that make you wonder what else they're getting wrong?)

Thankfully, the last few decades of neuroscience have given us stunning and fabulous news about the ability of the brain to rewire itself.

I'll name a few recommended books because that's what journalists like to do and because reading about the miracle that is our brain is much more fun than you might think.

The Brain That Changes Itself and *The Brain's Way of Healing* are two by Dr. Norman Doidge I found fascinating and actually bought for friends and family. *This Is Your Brain on Food* is a new one by a nutritional psychiatrist at Harvard named Dr. Uma Naidoo, digging deep into the life-changing link between your brain and your gut. And Daniel Amen's classic *Change Your Brain, Change Your Life* is smart, accessible, and plain-spoken.

"It is your brain that decides to get you out of bed in the morning to exercise, to give you a stronger, leaner body or to cause you to hit the snooze button and procrastinate your workout," he writes.

"Your brain is the command and control center of your body. If you want a better body, the first place to ALWAYS start is by having a better brain." Clear enough?

The latest research explains that the brain is beyond neuroplastic. It's *neuroevolving.* It can keep on growing and learning and making connections for eighty, ninety, one hundred years, or more. Even if you eat french fries.

An older brain is also a happier brain, if it's given proper care and attention, and I don't mean organic hair conditioner with added turmeric. Older brains can also be sharp, inquisitive, and optimistic to the end, or they can be compromised by mysterious conditions called Alzheimer's, senility, dementia—three of the scariest words in the English language, if you ask me.

So, let's ask another question: What can we humans do to keep our brains healthier and happier, more creative and less likely to crash as we come to the end of our road?

Here are some answers, all scientifically valid and evidence-based. You've probably heard them before but haven't yet included them in your self-care routine.

That's fine. It's never too late. Read through the following, and select one or two strategies that make sense to that big brain of yours. Then, take action!

Keep moving. The research is in, again and again: Physical activity is essential when it comes to growing your gray matter, particularly in those regions of the brain responsible for memory and higher-level thinking.

(An example of higher-level thinking would be tossing out all products with artificial sweeteners.)

According to a significant study published in the Journal of Alzheimer's Disease, brain scan studies now confirm what neuroscientists have been telling us for ages: Physical activity can prevent and postpone mental decline in aging brains. It can even substantially reduce the risk of Alzheimer's. Imagine that. No magic pills, no suspicious drugs. Just you and your body in motion, a few times a week.

And you'll be happy to know the brain researchers aren't talking about hardcore, super-strenuous workouts. Nope. Even recreational amounts of cycling, walking, and pulling weeds make a big difference when it comes to keeping you juiced and joyful, no matter your age.

Seek human contact. Social isolation deprives the brain of what it needs to thrive, which is why solitary confinement is used in prisons to punish people. And then there was COVID…and to some degree or another, we all suffered from the loneliness and lovelessness that happens when we don't get enough human contact, enough human touch.

We don't know when the next shutdown will happen in America, but for our brains and bodies to stay healthy, we have to be ready. We have to be proactive. We have to reach out to friends and family in ways that make our brains feel calm, not chaotic.

Enjoy brain breaks. Work smarter, not longer. Your brain works best when multitasking is limited or avoided and your amazing brain gets the time it needs to rest, to recall, to recalculate.

It's up to you to take brain breaks during your day, time away from the stress of the screen to walk, run, stretch, meditate, bike, dance, grow baby tomatoes, all admirable ways to let your brain relax and rejuvenate.

Nasal breathing will do that, too—talk about miracles—and so will getting enough sleep, at least seven or eight hours a night, in a dark room or wearing eyeshades, with your digital devices out of sight, out of mind.

Eat smart. I'm against the word "diet" as a verb, but there are certain types of diets-as-a-noun that are worth discussing.

One popular one for brain health is the MIND diet, developed by researchers at Rush University Medical Center in Chicago. The MIND diet is the love child of the DASH diet (recommended for lowering blood pressure) and the gold-standard Mediterranean diet. Besides whole grains, vegetables, and fruits, it also wants you to eat healthy fats such as salmon, nuts, and olive oil.

Why? Because they are the fats your body needs to stay in balance and combat inflammation. Nonfat products, which are mostly fake foods, don't do that. I know it's counterintuitive—as in, "Doesn't fat make you fat?"—but the bottom line is, nutrition-wise, you can't fool Mother Nature. Well, you can for a while, but she will probably mess with your brain and make you gain weight.

Your brain also loves leafy greens. Rush University researchers found that people who ate two servings a day had the cognitive ability of someone eleven years younger. Eleven years younger! Talk about nuts.

It's also crazy to think how much money the country could save if citizens were motivated and educated to eat real food instead of gobbling up the overprocessed foods that mess up our guts and help make our brains confused, chaotic, and malfunctioning.

"Alzheimer's is the most expensive disease in the country," says the Alzheimer's Association. "Every hour,

Alzheimer's costs the country $18.3 million. Today, Alzheimer's costs the country $236 billion a year and that will quadruple to more than $1 trillion over the next generation."

That blows my mind.

Control your devices. This is a toughie because, let's admit it, we are addicted to our devices. They were designed to addict us, and they've been successful beyond belief. Also more troubling. More and more, we can't live without them. And yet, living with them 24/7 is taking a toll on our brains that we're only beginning to understand.

Too much screen time—for business, for banking, for school, for socializing, for fun and games, for learning everything about everything—alters the very structure of your brain in ways that work against your well-being.

Brain scan research shows changes in your gray matter and changes in your white matter—and what really matters is how it's all linked to anxiety, depression, poorer concentration, and decreased impulse control, not to mention poor sleep, obesity, aggressive behaviors, and, for kids especially, unfortunate delays in social and emotional development.

With technology so tied into every fiber of our being, I don't expect our public health officials to start sounding the alarm anytime soon.

So, use your brain. Protect yourself from technology overload. Take time in your overly busy day to pry yourself away from all your distractive devices. Then, wander over to a quiet spot—indoors or out, in a chair or on a cushion—and meditate for some time.

ENERGY EXPRESS-O! Change Your Brain

"Meditation is not just blissing out under a mango tree. It completely changes your brain and therefore changes what you are."
—Matthieu Ricard

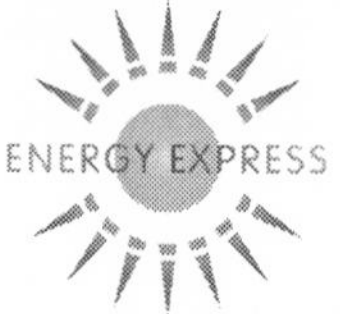

GOING DEEPER

Your brain wants to rewire itself into a happier, healthier state, but you have to help it. There are all sorts of brain activities you can do to stay sharper longer and live a more engaged, invigorated life. What are you willing to add to your self-care practice? What's a healthier brain worth to you?

Doing crossword puzzles makes you more skilled at doing crossword puzzles, and playing bridge makes you a better bridge player, and both can contribute to a healthier, happier brain.

But your brain grows best when you do new things in new ways. Learn sign language. Memorize a new poem every week. Take up a new sport. Brush your teeth with your nondominant hand. Travel to places you've never been. Take a different route home or to work.

Your brain likes it when new neural pathways are created, when synapses connect that never wired or fired together before.

Dancing—on your own, with a partner—can do that. So can curling up with a good book or pulling a mix of things out of your fridge and making something curiously edible for dinner.

Your brain thrives on challenge, on spontaneity, on the unpredictable. And if none of those are readily available, find the dark chocolate.

I've always been a shameless cheerleader for adventure travel. And I still walk the talk every chance I get. My longest, tallest, riskiest challenge was in 2000, an amazing, life-changing six-week trek through Nepal and Tibet that included a circumambulation of Mount Kailash—not the highest mountain in the world but said to be the holiest. The day the yak just ahead of me slipped off the trail and tumbled into the valley was a startling lesson in overcoming fear. (The yak survived. Me, too.) The continuing boom in adventure travel is one of the most thrilling healthy lifestyle trends of the last forty-five years, right up there with standing desks, nasal breathing, and the revolution in women's sports.

Explore Endlessly.

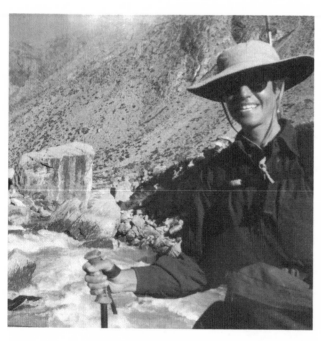

Show me a backpack and my toes start to tingle. I've been dog-sledding in Lapland, rafting in Costa Rica, bicycling in France, scuba diving in Mexico, sailing in Greece—I'll stop now—and the more adventures I take, the more enthusiastic I am about recommending them to others. Others being you, dear reader.

Why? Because active vacations are what joy feels like.

They are challenging, totally distracting, and sometimes life-changing. Best of all, they lure you into nature, where all the good stuff happens.

Mountains, rivers, forests—nature soothes and heals in a way that the blackjack tables at Caesar's Palace never can. When you challenge yourself outdoors—physically, mentally, emotionally—you discover new things about yourself. When I went around Mount Kailash, for instance, I learned I could take a pee in a plastic bag instead of crawling outside the tent into the bone-chilling cold and snow of 17,000 feet.

My favorite kind of adventure is the one I've never had before, which is why I leaped at the chance to go whale watching in winter in warm and sunny Baja, Mexico.

It wasn't just whale watching; it was amazingly close encounters with big blue whales, the largest animals to ever live on earth, even bigger than the dinosaurs.

And it wasn't just a time for deep breathing practice and oceanic meditation; it was time on the water with a wildly enthusiastic whale expert named, of all things, Michael Fishbach, founder of Eco-Interactions.

"These guys are a complete mystery," Michael says about his pals, the big blues, after more than twenty years of research. "Why do they keep coming back to Baja? When do they give birth? And where? There's so much we really don't know."

What we do know about the big blue whales is mind-boggling. They weigh up to 150 tons. The heart of a blue whale is the size of a Volkswagen beetle, and their arteries are large enough for a child to crawl through. They can swim at speeds up to thirty miles per hour, can dive down to 10,000 feet, and can hold their breath up to an hour. The average length is seventy to eighty-five feet, but they can grow to one hundred feet or more. Their life span is thought to be sixty to seventy years. They eat up to four tons of krill a day—tiny, shrimp-like creatures—hold the cocktail sauce.

Here's the sad part: They are a seriously endangered species. Thanks to illegal whaling, pollution, fishing nets, cargo ships, and killer whales, there are only about 10,000 blue whales left on the planet, which is why Michael and some colleagues started the Great Whale Conservancy under the umbrella of Earth Island Institute.

You can do your part by visiting the Earth Island Institute website and learning about his campaign, but the best way to get a feeling for what magnificent beasts they are is to do what I was lucky enough to do and go out with Michael at six in the morning on the Sea of Cortez—with the full moon setting on one side of the bay and the fiery Mexican sun rising on the other. And watch for spouts. And just listen.

"HHH-A-A-AUhhhh!" is my lame attempt to repeat a sound I'll never forget—the exhalation of a big blue whale rising to the surface to take a breath. Wow. How can I explain? The blues have a *presence.*

Energetically, you feel a mysterious connection to an extraordinary being. When they fluke—their huge tails rising high in the air as they slide into the sea—it feels like a blessing. Blues are notoriously calm and trusting, neither threatened nor threatening, and their brains function on a higher level than many of our elected officials.

Some of the twenty to thirty blue whales we saw came within fifteen feet of our little boat. So close! I gasped in amazement. I imagined myself on their backs, diving deep into my own fears of the sea. I felt inexplicably overwhelmed with joy and gratitude. This never happened to me at Disney World.

ENERGY EXPRESS-O! Find Your Inner Traveler

"If you think adventure is dangerous, try routine; it's lethal."—Paulo Coelho

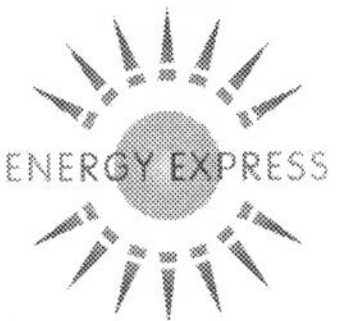

GOING DEEPER

How many travel plans did you have to cancel when COVID-19 shut the world down?

Me, too. What can we do? Adapt and survive. The past is the past. And in the future? Who knows what travel will look like.

All the more reason to sit down and dream up your ideal adventure vacation. I can't say what it is for you, but for me, it involves a new tent, a sleeping bag, and a small solar charger. I'm still filling in the details.

So, what revs up your engines? Fishing in Wisconsin? Biking on the back roads of Oregon? Renting an RV and heading out to whatever patch of natural beauty calls to you?

If you can dream it, you can plan it. If you don't, who will?

And remember this: The best adventures begin when you let go of what's holding you back. If you're afraid to commit to some form of adventure travel, considering COVID and all the restrictions you think are necessary, sit with that and examine your hesitation. Don't abandon caution or common sense, but allow yourself to err on the side of bravery and adventure. In other words, live your life.

When you return home from whatever trip you took, go

through your photos, and make a book. Include your feelings and fears, your trials and triumphs.

What challenges appeared, and how did you meet them?
When were the best parts? The hard parts?
What did you learn?
Where are you going next year?

Meditation is trendy. Meditation is cool. Meditation in the workplace. Meditation in school. (I feel like I'm channeling Dr. Seuss.) So, here's my question: Is meditation part of your practice? If ever there was a time to say yes, it's now, during and after the time of COVID-19. Meditation makes the unknowable less unsettling, the terrifying less traumatic. Reading about it won't calm you, but experiencing it will. It's not a maybe; it's a sure thing, scientifically proven time and time again. The only way to fail is to give up on yourself, which you are less likely to do after I introduce you to the work of a well-known meditation master, Sharon Salzberg. I've described her as a cross between Melissa McCarthy and the Dalai Lama, and I mean that in the nicest, kindest way.

Meditate on This.

Before *Real Happiness*, Sharon Salzberg's book about creating a more joyful life, she experienced real unhappiness and deep despair.

Her father left home when she was four. Her mother died when she was nine. She went to live with her grandparents, but her grandfather died soon after. Her father returned, tried to kill himself, and ended up a mental patient for the rest of his life. And you think you had a tough childhood?

By the time Sharon left for college, she'd lived in five different households, all chaotic and confusing. She felt abandoned and angry. And then, when she was eighteen—convinced she was unworthy of love—Sharon went to India. And her life changed in wonderful ways.

Sharon learned to meditate, to look deep within. And what she discovered is what she's been living and teaching ever since: that goodness exists in everyone, that she is wildly worthy of love, that everyone deserves to be happy, and that everyone can be happy, once you learn to be mindful, compassionate, and free of judgment.

"If you can breathe, you can meditate," she writes in *Real Happiness: The Power of Meditation*, a terrific how-to guide that includes audio of Sharon's sultry tones, expertly narrating nine guided meditations.

As co-founder of the Insight Meditation Society, she's been teaching her style of Buddhist-based meditation for more than thirty-five years, and in this book, her eighth, she's stripped away all the esoteric Buddhist text and terms and gone straight to the heart of the teachings. "Once we have a sense of a center," she writes, "we can more easily withstand the onslaught of overstimulation, uncertainty and anxiety the world launches at us, without getting overwhelmed."

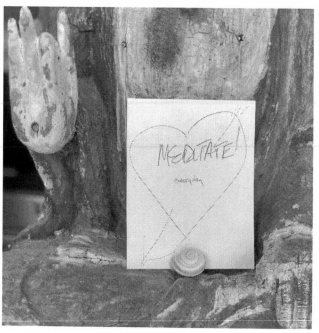

I heard Sharon explore the power of meditation at a Real Happiness retreat at the Upaya Institute and Zen Center in Santa Fe, New Mexico. It's a think tank for going beyond thinking, and the founder, Joan Halifax Roshi, my friend of many years, has a well-deserved reputation for presenting world-class teachers.

Sharon fits the bill. She's funny, smart, and a gifted

storyteller, with a soothing voice and surprisingly sleepy eyes. Her no-big-deal, anyone-can-do-it approach to meditation is gentle, inviting, and entirely profound.

If you want to learn, or you're curious to know what's involved, Sharon has come up with a twenty-eight-day program, step by step, story by story, breath by breath. Without judgment, and with humor, she points the way toward a life of compassion, connection, and loving kindness, while teaching the skills to let go of fear, anger, and envy.

At the end of day one, I bought three copies of her book for friends.

(I could have bought thirty.)

Here are a few highlights from her talks:

Meditation isn't a religion. You don't have to be Buddhist or Hindu or a yogi to practice. The techniques Sharon teaches can be done within any faith tradition or be done in an entirely secular way. You don't need special skills or a huge chunk of time every day. (She recommends twenty minutes, but if you've only got five, start there.)

Meditation is not an attempt to stop thinking, she says. It's "a way to recognize our thoughts, to observe and understand them, and relate to them more skillfully."

Why practice meditation? Meditation is a medical miracle. Clinical studies show it promotes wellness, reduces stress, boosts learning and memory, improves sleep and depression, lowers blood pressure, and much more. Sharon focuses more on the emotional and psychological benefits: learning how to stay in the moment, letting go of judgments, becoming aware of a calm and stable center that gets us through tough times.

Meditation isn't passive, she says. "Deepening our concentration brings us power and energy and healing."

Losing focus is normal. Sharon's taught thousands of

people to meditate, and the one truth we all need to hear, over and over, is that losing concentration is normal. It happens to everyone. You start out focusing on your breath, and after just a few inhales and exhales, you're thinking about lunch or your itchy nose or a new app for organizing all your other apps. No problem, says Sharon. Just start over again, without a moment of shame or frustration.

And what if you feel bored, restless, deep sadness when you attempt to meditate?

"A difficult session is just as valuable as a pleasant one—maybe more so," she knows. "We can look mindfully at joy, sorrow or anguish. It doesn't matter what's going on; transformation comes from changing our relationship to what's going on."

It's as simple as that. Ha!

ENERGY EXPRESS-O! Let Go of the Struggle

"Your goal is not to battle with the mind,
but to witness the mind."
—Swami Muktananda

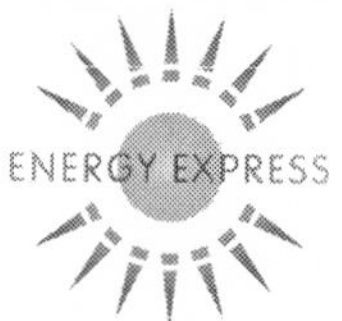

GOING DEEPER

There are many paths to a meditation practice. You probably know all of them: classes, apps, gifted teachers, millions of books. And all of them lead to one simple behavior.

Sit.

If your body can sit comfortably on a cushion in a classic, cross-legged posture, go for it. It's impressive, but not necessary.

Being impressive is also not necessary.

If you prefer to sit quietly on a chair or a kneeling stool, that's fine, too.

Start where you are.

Close your eyes; draw your awareness inside; and examine your ideas about meditation.

Don't judge. Don't react to every sensation. Just be curious.

Do you think it's all hocus-pocus? And boring?

You can think that, no problem, and then come back to the sound of your breath.

Meditate on whatever thoughts and feelings arise. Positive and negative, all thoughts are welcome. If nothing arises, just try not to fall asleep.

If you fall asleep, so what? Smile. Who doesn't love a little nap?

After a while, slowly open your eyes, and congratulate yourself for finding the time to sit.

Don't worry about whether you did this little exercise right.

Just doing it is doing it right.

Come back tomorrow.

Self-care is the best care; I've been saying it for years. But now I really mean it. The COVID crisis revealed what a sick country we are, and we are paying a horrible price. Why did America lead the way in the early days, with the highest number of infections and deaths? Because our dear citizens were so unhealthy to begin with! We've been living with an inefficient, inadequate, discriminatory, who-cares-about-prevention health care system far too long. It's working for pharmaceutical and insurance companies, but it's delivering early death and disease to too many of our friends and family members. America is ranked about thirty-fifth among nations when it comes to our citizens' health and well-being. Cuba is thirtieth; Chile is thirty-third. Life expectancy is going down in the U.S., while obesity, diabetes, and suicides are going up. So, what to do? Get the best medical care you can; at the same time, educate yourself, and practice intentional self-care. The fact that you're reading this book means you've already begun.

Take Care of Yourself.

"If I am not for myself, who will be for me?" said Hillel the Elder, a wise teacher who lived in Jerusalem around the time B.C. became A.D.

That's the essence of self-care. It's not selfish; it's sensible. And it's particularly sensible in the time of a global pandemic, when our overworked, underfunded public health officials say everything about face masks and social distancing, and almost nothing about prevention strategies that can strengthen your body's own defense system and make you less likely to get sick.

When you decide to be in charge of your own health and wellness—being active, eating real food, getting enough sleep, doing practices that calm your mind and boost your immune system—everyone you know, including your pets, will benefit. And yes, your risk of succumbing to COVID-19 can substantially reduce.

Hillel, again: "Take care of yourself. You never know when the world will need you."

And now the hop, skip, and a jump to injury prevention because that's one great way we can practice self-care. Physical activity without body awareness is going to lead to injuries if you're not careful and, often, even if you are. Without knowing why or how, we wreck our lower backs, tear our shoulders, strain our knees, and the cost in terms of health care dollars spent and work hours lost is crippling.

As a self-caring person, there is a lot you can do to avoid sports injuries. Sure, accidents will happen—you fall off your bike, the curb, the wagon—but the more you understand the basics of self-care, the prouder Hillel will be of you.

Don't overdo it. Overuse injuries are the most common sports injuries. They pop up in different disguises—back pain, sore shins, strained knees—but the cause is the same: You're doing too much, too soon, with a body that isn't strong, aligned, or flexible enough to take the stress. You have to back off to move forward. And if you're working with a bully of a trainer who pushes you too hard, screaming, "No pain, no gain," get yourself a more evolved coach.

Develop body awareness. Pretend I'm shaking your shoulders now because this is so important. To lower your risk of injury—any injury—learn some basic anatomy so that you can sense your body, listen to your body, even talk back to your body, giving new meaning to "I've Got You Under My Skin."

Working with this felt sense of body awareness—Is my sacrum pulling to the right? Am I engaging my diaphragm when I breathe in and out of my nose? Why can't I widen the spaces between my toes?—puts you on a path to personal well-being in a way that nothing else can. Really!

So before you put yourself in motion—at play, at work—take a few moments to scan your whole body, from the top of your cranium to the bottom of your corns.

When you sense tension—a stiff neck, tight shoulders, hips that hurt when you walk—relax and release, a mind-body trick that is easier said than done but always worth the effort. Then use your mind's eye to bathe the area with fresh, revitalizing breath.

This concept of tuning into your inner self may sound mysterious, but it's not. It's solid science, the essence of prevention, but we're not taught it, and our Western-trained doctors don't encourage it. Qigong, yoga, meditation, mindfulness, and somatics training can lead you in that direction, and so can a terrific book I'm constantly reading called *Awakening Somatic Intelligence* by Risa F. Kaparo, Ph.D. Fascinating!

Slow down. If you're concerned about getting hurt playing sports, know it's okay to slow down. Slow walking. Conscious running. You don't have to go fast to get into shape, physically or mentally.

The fact is when you slow down your movement, you have time to zone in on what's going on with your muscles, your joints, your breath…and it's this feedback that tells you when to ease off and when to speed up.

If you can nip a body injury in the bud—before it ends up needing a doctor, tests, drugs—you save yourself a whole lot of aggravation, money, and stress.

Focus and breathe. If your mind wanders and you lose focus when you work out—pondering the past, worrying about the future, texting in between—painful accidents happen more easily.

Listening to your breath can help keep you focused. Learn to breathe fully, rhythmically, and, most important because it's been ignored for too long, learn to breathe in and out of your nose, not your mouth. Not only will a focus on nasal breathing lower your risk of injury, but it's also a good way to release tension and create stability so your body can move more easily, with greater flow.

The opposite of conscious breathing is holding your breath. It's a complete no-no for any sport. And it's especially risky when it comes to lifting and lowering heavy weights because it can push your blood pressure way too high.

Balance your workout. Muscle imbalance—strong quads but weak hamstrings, a ripped ten-pack in front but tightness and weakness in your lower back—is a common cause of sports injuries. Learn to work your body in a balanced way, front and back, side to side, top to bottom.

Check your gear. Sometimes, sports injuries result from a mismatch between you and your equipment: a bike seat that's too low, a tennis racket that's too heavy, ten-year-old running shoes. Your gear should support and fit your body. If you suspect it doesn't, talk to an expert to make sure you're not setting yourself up for injuries down the line.

ENERGY EXPRESS-O! Why Self-Care is a Must

"The 34 countries that are ahead of the U.S. in the Bloomberg health rankings all offer universal health care to their people. This means that preventive, primary and acute care is available to 100% of the population. In contrast, 25-35 million Americans do not have health care insurance, and an equal number are underinsured."

—Etienne Deffarges

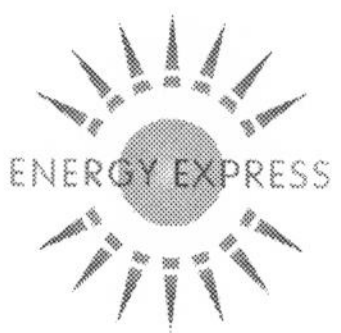

GOING DEEPER

Anatomy is destiny, Freud said. He was probably wrong about a bunch of stuff, but he was right on target with that. If you don't know and sense your anatomy—where your body parts are placed and how they work together—you are destined for a very rough ride through our broken health care system.

Learning a bit about your own anatomy is an unusual but highly effective way to promote your own health and healing.

You don't have to memorize anything. You are your own final exam.

Just explore and embrace a big-picture understanding of where your vital organs are, including your heart, your lungs, your kidneys, your colon.

Investigate the exquisite architecture of your body, including major bones, vital tendons and ligaments, more than six hundred muscles. Learn how your body is constructed, connected, and how it works.

All the while, learn to listen to your body. Talk to it, too. Sensation is the language of the body. You are a living electric grid, and the flow of energy, or the stuckness you feel, is your body communicating to you.

Tune in, even though your doctor may never mention this as something useful. It is. If you feel jumpy or joyful, tight or terrific, your body is telling you something you need to hear.

Don't judge; don't be scared; just pay attention, and be curious enough to figure out what might be going on. If your doctor is totally dismissive of this approach to self-care, please find another doctor.

Knowing your anatomy will help you befriend your body in a way that makes personal well-being possible. Your body is a mystery and a miracle, and the sooner you start a dialogue, the sooner you will be taking charge, making change, nurturing body and mind with your breath.

I am certain Hillel would approve.

How you age matters. There are zillions of books out there to help you age gracefully, wildly, mindfully, with or without Botox. But what about de-aging, what Kazuaki Tanahashi calls the "Miracle of Each Moment"? Kaz has inspired me time and time again with his gorgeous calligraphy and his boundless enthusiasm for painting, poetry, and peace. He's ageless, I remember thinking soon after we met. And now I know why.

Practice De-Aging.

I have a friend visiting me on this small, remote Greek island where I live several months a year. He is a Zen teacher, translator, artist, author, and world-class peace activist. His name is Kazuaki Tanahashi. Sometimes, when people say to him, "Hello. How are you?" Kaz will laugh and answer, "I am de-aging."

In his eighties now, Kaz is the inventor of de-aging. It's not a product or a program. It's a concept, a way of slowing down the aging process without resorting to desperate anti-aging measures involving pills, plastic surgery, or genetic re-engineering.

"Anti-aging is defensive thinking," Kaz explains to me one day after breakfast, sitting in our room with a view, overlooking the Aegean sea. "De-aging is more active. Each moment, we have a choice."

Kaz takes a breath, and so do I. I've heard him talk about de-aging before. This time, I'm taking notes.

"The idea is we lose vitality and gain vitality each moment. Aging is not a one-way street, going downhill. We become older, we become younger, every moment."

Kaz has explained his quantum physics-based de-aging theory to many friends who are doctors, and they all agree it's a good one.

"We age as a whole," Kaz continues, his long scraggly beard waving in the breeze. "Our body, our mind...we can't reverse it. But when we look at aging at the micro level—each day, each hour, each moment—we see that it goes up and down. So in each moment, we have a choice."

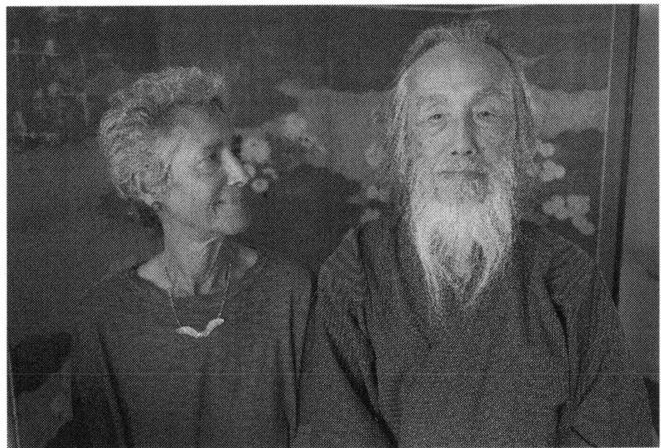

The choice is between doing something that ages us or de-ages us, something that makes us more vital or less vital, more healthy or less healthy.

He mentions eating well and exercising. (I feel a wellness column writing itself in my mind, which means I'll be free to spend the afternoon de-aging at my favorite beach. I am choosing to be happy.)

"If I'm tired, I can choose to take a walk, or I can watch TV," he elaborates. "I can choose to relax and meditate, or I can smoke. I can overwork, or I can rest. I can take a job that is more stressful or less stressful...and in this way, we can shape our life. Are we aging, or are we de-aging? It's an active choice."

When it comes to living a healthier, happier lifestyle, it always comes down to personal choices.

Fortunately for all of us, you don't have to be a Zen master to figure it out. Will you have a donut and diet cola for breakfast or oatmeal, walnuts, and maple syrup? Hold onto anger or let it go? Choose to drive or walk or bike?

"You can't really control overall aging," Kaz says, "but by doing de-aging, we can slow it down."

"So de-aging is a kind of practice," I say. Kaz doesn't pick up on the word "practice." I feel myself aging, just a little.

"What are some other ways we can de-age?" I ask.

"It's important to be excited about life!" Kaz says, raising his voice to just above a whisper. "Being in love! You could be in love with art, grandchildren, or doing service work. Have a passion. Love what you do!"

Kaz says he loves what he does—writing, painting, running a revolutionary nonprofit called A World Without Armies—but he is aware of his tendency to do too much for too long.

"I am Japanese; I'm a kind of workaholic. I have to tell myself to slow down, to be lazy. Lazy people don't have to be reminded to be lazy." He stops to laugh at his own joke. "To be lazy doesn't mean not to work. It means to slow down, do less work, and be more effective. That kind of laziness."

Negative emotions get in the way of de-aging, Kaz goes on. "Anger, envy, jealousy, hatred…all these negative emotions contribute to aging. So you have to find a way to turn a negative situation into something positive. This is the practice of being calm, more compassionate, more understanding. This turns aging into de-aging."

It's time to take a break, another form of de-aging practice. Can I call it a practice even if Kaz does not?

It's something to think about as I sit on the sand, building a tower out of beach stones, slowly balancing one little rock on another, watching myself grow younger every moment.

ENERGY EXPRESS-O! Zen and Now

"Be open to all teachers, and all teachings,
and listen with your heart."
—Ram Dass

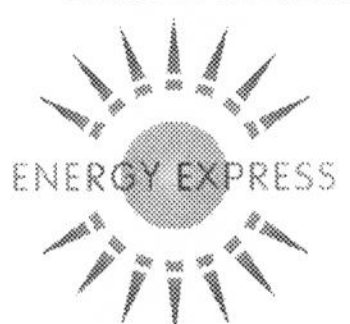

GOING DEEPER

If de-aging is your goal—and better living through chemistry isn't—what will you choose to do differently?

The examples below are only examples. They just lie there like useless suggestions on a meaningless page, unless they spark something inside of you, something you are motivated to make happen. That's the only way change will happen. Duh.

So, consider some of these de-aging possibilities:

—Turn off your cell phone at mealtime.

—Rescue a dog, and take it for walks twice a day.

—Slow down.

—Give up road rage, name-calling, blaming the Other.

—Get more sleep.

—Join a local singing group.

—Tutor a child.

—Work less; play more. No guilt allowed.

—Take every single day and moment of your vacation.

—_____________ (fill in the blank).

De-aging is all about the choices you make, every day, day by day, day in, day out.

And then you die.

SPRING

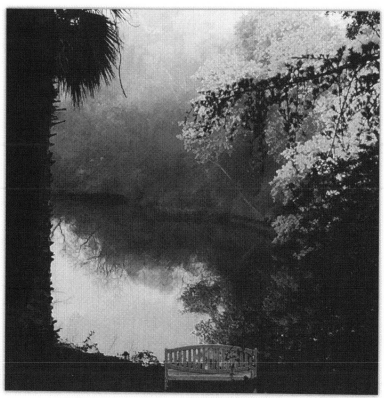

Napa, California

"This spring wakes us, nurtures us, revitalizes us.
How often does your spring come?"
—Gary Zukav

"Never yet was a springtime,
when the buds forgot to bloom."
—Margaret Elizabeth Sangster

"Spring has returned. The Earth is like a
child who knows poems."
—Rainer Maria Rilke

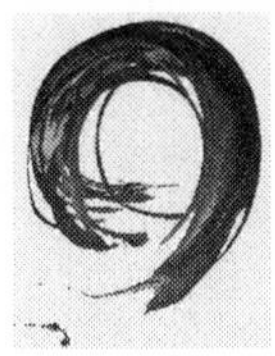

When the seasons change, so can we. It's true for every season, but it's especially true in spring, when all things blossom and grow. The pandemic was catastrophic, no question, but it helped us focus on what we personally need to blossom and grow. You can spring forward in your own life by staying positive, setting small doable goals, sticking with your plan, and, nicest of all, being kind to yourself and others, including the annoying, unsupportive others. For many years, I've been training myself to eat more slowly, chew more consciously. It's a battle; I'm still the first one finished. I'm a work in progress, I tell myself. Someday, if it's important to me, I'll chew with more awareness. It's not that big a deal. All is well.

Spring Forward.

"Springtime is in the air," writes Kenneth Cohen, a Qigong master of the Tao. "A good time for spring cleaning of mind and body through meditation, healing practices, eating spring greens, drinking herbal tonics, and bathing in natural hot springs."

Before I shower you with my own suggestions about how to celebrate spring, let me ask: What's your number one wish when it comes to living a healthier life?

Think for a minute. We're not in a rush.

The truth is, we humans can make positive change any day—if we're really ready. But in spring, Mother Nature gives us an extra cellular push.

Spring is the time of new beginnings, new growth. In spring, when all things made of light turn toward the light, it's easier for you to do the same.

Consider these five ways to get your sap rising:

Do something you're afraid to do. Fear can keep us from being the person we'd like to become. Over the next few weeks and months, face a fear…and work through it.

Volunteer at a hospice. Stop coloring your hair. Jump out of a plane, with an instructor, tandem, screaming.

When we overcome a fear, our whole body relaxes into a feeling of confidence and well-being. If I can do the thing I feared, what else can I do?

Look into your biochemistry. Face the facts. Most doctors know next to nothing about nutrition. It's lack of training more than lack of interest, I hope, but it means you have to make the effort yourself to figure out what foods, vitamins, and supplements you need. Your nutritional profile—your biochemistry—is uniquely your own. Just because your best friend takes iron or vitamin B-12 shots doesn't mean you should. The best strategy is to have basic bloodwork done and find a nutritionist who will analyze the results to determine what you personally need—and what you don't.

Remember: Real food—unprocessed, locally grown, mostly organic—is the smartest way to serve your body what it needs. Supplements are always second, and they should only be taken as necessary, not because they are being promoted online or at your health food store.

Step up your physical activity. Most people insist they'd like to exercise more—more walking! more biking!—but at the end of the day, they claim they don't have the time. Horse feathers. In reality, you *make* the time. You organize your day so there is time. This spring, stop making excuses, and start organizing. If it means fewer hours on social media, congratulations.

A few more ideas spring to mind: Get up thirty to sixty minutes earlier—to walk, to practice nasal breathing, to move your body in ways that feel good. Take the stairs instead of elevators and escalators. Keep a sturdy stationary bike next to the TV, and sprint your way through every dopey commercial that pushes drugs with side effects so serious they require other drugs to treat them. Good for business, bad for public health.

This spring, no matter how many times you've failed to make physical activity a priority, begin again. Plan for success, and celebrate in the summer with something you really want, like an e-bike, a stand-up desk, time to just be, not do.

Find your stress, and let it go. Stress happens. Before, during, and after the pandemic, stress was, is, and will always be with us. Some amount of stress is good for the body, it's true. More true is that the stress you're feeling is often overwhelming—too much, too often, too linked to sickness and disease. So, to stay healthy, you need to have a strategy, a practice you enjoy, a practice that keeps the stress from making you unwell.

Choose an activity that lowers stress, heightens awareness, lightens anxiety, and feels like joy. Meditation? Cooking? Stand-up yoga on paddleboards?

Health experts agree that more than seventy-five percent of all sickness and disease is related to stress, in your body and in your mind. That's an astonishing number.

This spring, find it in your body, and let it go.

Eat smart. Turn over a new leaf this spring—preferably spinach, kale, or arugula—and swear off processed foods. That will be a huge boost to your immune system, giving you one more layer of defense against incoming viruses and bacteria of all sorts, including COVID and its cousins to follow.

Give your kitchen a spring cleaning—a mindful makeover. Read labels. If the so-called food has line after line of ingredients you can't pronounce, toss it. And sugar? Cut back; cut down; and keep eliminating it, one piece of pie at a time.

If you wean yourself off sugar this spring, you'll sail through summer with a lightness and a brightness you've never known before.

ENERGY EXPRESS-O! How To Be Successful

"May your choices reflect your hopes, not your fears."
—Nelson Mandela

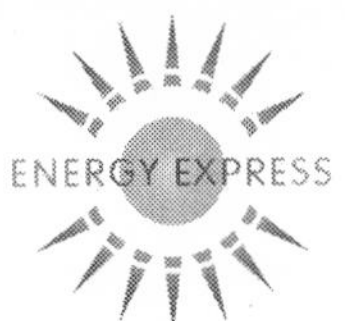

GOING DEEPER

Buy a notebook, and write down the change you want to see for yourself this spring.

Why is this change important to you?

How will you make it happen?

Write down the details of your practice, and keep track of your progress, focusing on the positive every step of the way. If you slip-slide away for a day or a week, accept it, appreciate your rebellious nature, and get back to your journal.

Journaling is to personal well-being what wheels are to a car. It moves you forward at the same time it helps you focus your energy and awareness so you can reflect on how things are going.

If you keep your journal in one place you visit every day—next to your toothbrush, under your keys—you are a thousand times more likely to write in it.

Maybe keeping a journal won't work for you. But maybe it will. It did for me. I was a much heavier person, a junior size 15-16, when I graduated high school.

My first journal was my path to changing the way I ate, and your journal can steer you in the direction you decide to go, keeping track to stay on track.

What do you have to lose?

Fear is nature's way of helping us grow. Fear holds us back from doing lots of stuff, until we overcome fear, and then we realize what a friend and ally it is. When I was young, I feared I'd never get over my stutter. How long will I b-b-b-b-be like this? How can I t-t-t talk in class? Marry a guy named P-P-P-Preston!? Over time, my stutter went away. Other fears followed—I used to go crazy when I'd see a spider—but now I have a point of view. And when I take that point of view on vacation, well, it leads to unforgettable experiences.

Make Your Getaway.

I've been a cheerleader for adventure travel since the first time I jumped on my bicycle and yelled, "Giddyup!" What's ahead, around the corner, up the trail? Who will I meet? What will I see? Why am I here?

My curiosity about the unexplored and unpredictable has led me to trekking in Tibet, kayaking down the Wisconsin River, hiking in the Rockies, and hut-to-hut cross-country skiing in Vermont. (After only two lessons. Oy.)

Recently, I set a course I'd never been on before: sailing.

I'm actually a bit afraid of the sea. (It's wet, and there are all those unseen creatures lurking below. Ick.) But that didn't stop me from saving up and signing on for seven nights of sailing with friends in the small Cycladic islands of the Aegean, all doing our charter best to help Greece out of a devastating economic crisis she did not deserve.

Adventure travel, on the other hand, is something we all deserve. It's fun. It's challenging. It's mystical enough to teach you lessons you need to learn, and it has the potential to change your life in ways that five days at Disney World just can't.

Where you go isn't as important as planning an adventure that calls to you—whatever, wherever, whenever. You're never too old to be brave. All you need is the willingness to step out of your comfort zone and, in this case, onto the deck of a sweet fifty-year-old fifty-six-foot ketch with three cozy guest cabins and a magnificent and joyful master captain willing to take us wherever the wind and our seasickness would allow (www.patmosailing.com).

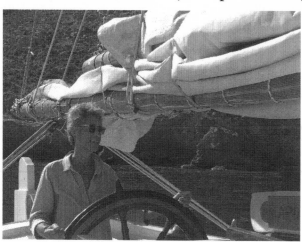

Sailing is a sport. I wasn't sure it was before my week at sea, but now I know for sure: Sailing is real work, physically and mentally. Whereas watching *other* people sail is a perpetual dream. There are mainsails and jibs to be raised, lines to be pulled, anchors to be set.

And more than brute strength and a strong back, you need focus. Total focus and intense concentration—and that's just for walking around the deck. Sailboats are loaded with lines, pulleys, fairleads, and steel rigging tracks that sit there, waiting to snag any passing toe that isn't paying attention.

All of which led me to one of the great lessons learned on board, a teaching I keep hurrying back to: slow down; take your time; stay in the moment. And get ice on that toe lickety-split.

Pack light. Adventure travel requires you to lay out the stuff you need for the trip and then leave half of it at home. Sailboats are all about storage, and the lack of it, so you have to make do with less. And having a strict sense of order will give you extra room to store more goodies, like sea salt potato chips and Greek butter cookies.

I know it sounds shallow, but one of the things I loved most about my first sailing journey was discovering I could wear the same shorts and T-shirt day after day and nobody cared, least of all me. I had that liberating insight on the tiny island of Despotiko, walking around the spectacular ruins of a 2,500-year-old temple of Apollo and Artemis, and by golly, I thanked them.

Stay active. Sailing involves a lot of sitting. Sitting and reading; sitting and eating; sitting and staring at clouds that suddenly take on the shape of Mrs. Blum, my seventh-grade math teacher. All worthwhile activities, but thank Neptune I brought my yoga mat. Swim, stretch, float…just don't sit, sit, sit. Find ways to keep your body juiced and open and your mind will follow.

Go with the flow. In nature, there is a divinely natural tendency to feel very small and very large at the same time. Being at sea, under the stars, brings wave after wave of realization that you are a tiny speck in an incomprehensibly deep universe, so there's no point in being anything but grateful for the life you have.

ENERGY EXPRESS-O! To Sail Is to Surrender

"That's what sailing is, a dance, and your partner is the sea. She's the leader, not you. You and your boat are dancing to her tune."

—Michael Morpurgo

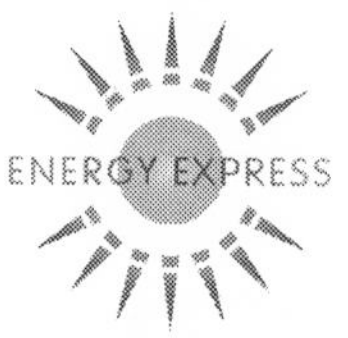

GOING DEEPER

One Sunday morning, at the peak of the first COVID shutdown, I woke up, had my breakfast, stood in front of my computer, and went to Rwanda, a small, hilly, spectacularly scenic nation in the heart of Africa.

It was my first virtual travel adventure—a live-streaming event produced by Steppin' Out Adventures—and it won't be my last.

Is it as thrilling as being there? No. Real adventure travel can't be faked. But did I experience enough of the Rwandan culture, music, and dance, not to mention some native Rwandans, to make it feel like a fun and foreign adventure? Absolutely.

Rwanda is a country of about 13 million people, with five volcanoes, twenty-three lakes, dense tropics, many wild rivers, and, of course, the mountain gorillas made famous by Dian Fossey.

"There is so much more to Rwanda than the gorillas," host Greg told my Zoom group of twenty-four during our two hours together. He's the founder of the Red Rocks Initiative, a community-led center for conservation, tourism, and art, and Greg was happy to introduce us to his team of Rwandan drummers and dancers, who played the music and sang the songs that are so much a part of their history and culture.

It was a completely interactive experience, in real time, nighttime in Rwanda and daytime for us. The Rwandans told us their names, and we told them ours. Some women showed us their handmade drums and demonstrated different beats. We showed them three feet of snow and asked about their paintings. And we all joined in on a traditional Rwandan country song called "Dushengeye Turimba," which roughly translates into, "We are standing before you, singing with happiness."

For more information about virtual adventure travel, and the real kind, too, take a look at SteppinOutAdventures.com. The founder and executive director is someone I've known and admired for years, Robin Richman. And if you tell her I sent you—use the code Dod Brad—she might offer you a family discount.

Now I have a miraculous little garden, but for years, I could only relish the possibility. I loved to listen to people who watered their curly endive and ate their own arugula and grew sweet basil on their back porch. "It's my meditation," one friend confided, and I swooned with a bad case of greens envy. And flowers! What's more beautiful than a vase filled with saucer-sized roses from your own yard? But beware. Gardening can be a source of pain if you don't know beans about preventing injuries. Your most personal fitness trainer offers up a short-course on growing your awareness.

Dig Into Nature.

Are you into gardening? Please say yes. Food you grow yourself tastes better, costs less, has greater nutritional value, AND leaves a carbon footprint the size of a grape. It's a kind of miracle. I can't think of a mean thing to say about it, except…

Gardening isn't an aerobic sport, and it won't grow your fitness the way running, walking, and biking will. But it sure can produce lots of pleasure, not to mention Green Goddess cauliflower, Box Car Willie tomatoes, and Purple Passion asparagus.

Gardening also helps you cultivate a calm, focused mind while you're putting all the major muscles of your body to work—digging, lifting, and carrying. Besides burning calories, gardening connects us to the earth, and it's that mindful exchange of energy—you plant; nature grows—that is so joyful and satisfying.

Growing stuff in a garden is also a splendid way to plant ideas in your child's brain about what real food is and how good it can taste. Next thing you know, your ten-year-old is snacking on kale chips instead of corn chips, and he goes to sleep at night dreaming of broccoli stalks the size of baseball bats.

Well, not immediately, but over time. Tending to a little garden—even a flowerpot on the windowsill—can give your child a wondrous sense of being connected to nature. It's a good thing.

Gardening is right up there with fly-fishing as a low-injury activity. But you still need awareness. If you rush into your garden chores carelessly, tweeting and texting, your mind a million miles away, you can wrench your back, create crippling tension in your shoulders, or wind up with a neck stiffer than a newborn zucchini.

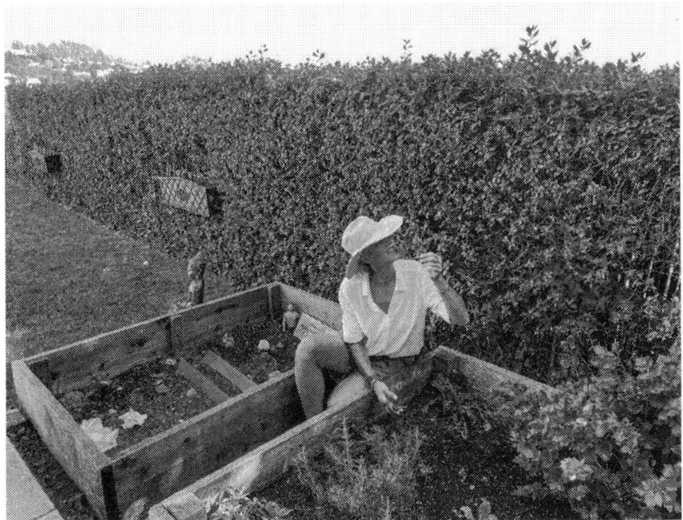

So, before you start growing a list of gardening aches and pains, consider the following:

Learn to lift and carry. Prepare before you lift. Take a breath or two, and make sure your body is aligned and ready. Relax your head and neck, and drop your shoulders. When you lift, engage your core muscles (your abs, glutes, torso muscles on both sides of your spine, front and back). Lift slowly, pushing down through your feet and drawing up through your legs. No grabbing and snatching, and no undue pressure or strain on your lower back.

Carry heavy items (bags of fertilizers, rocks, prize-winning watermelons) close to your body, not out in front of you, arms outstretched. Give thanks for the wheelbarrow, and use one whenever you feel like it.

And finally, think it through before you do. If you think something is too heavy to lift or carry by yourself, it probably is. Macho is not an evolved state. Get help, and avoid a nasty injury.

Small bites avoid big problems. When you shovel or dig, be content to take small bites with good tools that fit your hand. Good gloves will protect those hands, so find a pair you like, even if they're pink.

And just like in the gym, don't overdo it. Big shovels loaded with heavy dirt can easily strain your back, shoulders, and knees.

To avoid post-planting strains and sprains, keep your mind focused on the task at hand: smaller loads, no sudden twisting or torquing, moving with awareness so you stay balanced and aligned.

A little protection goes a long way. Start with your knees. Protect their delicate structure by kneeling on a foam pad or towels. Protect your eyes with sunglasses and a hat. Protect your skin from the burning sun with a proper cover-up—clothes or nontoxic sunscreen—and by moderating exposure.

Begin your gardening with a little warmup, simple range-of-motion stretches that juice up your joints and energize your muscles for the work ahead. If you feel pain when you garden, back off, relax, and, if you start up again, look for an easier way to do the same task. Drink enough water to stay hydrated, and don't stay in any position too long.

Cultivate calmness. To make all your gardening chores more effortless, move with the flow of your breath. This can work wonders in all your activities, from shooting baskets to unloading your car. Focusing on your breath gets you started, but then it's up to you to immerse yourself in the moment and not distract yourself with memories of the past or worries for the future.

Growth sustains life. What's good for the plants is good for you, too. Once that seed is planted, you'll never want to buy another plastic box of tasteless tomatoes again.

ENERGY EXPRESS-O! Peas and Prosperity

"Everything that slows us down and forces patience, everything that sets us back into the slow circles of nature, is a help. Gardening is an instrument of grace."
—May Sarton

ENERGY EXPRESS

GOING DEEPER

When the global pandemic planted fear in every household, millions of people started to tend to their gardens. This week, join in. Do something related to growing food.

If you don't have room for a garden, plant a window box, and fill it with the herbs of your choice. Parsley, mint, basil, and rosemary will give you a taste of success with very little effort.

And your dinner guests will go crazy when they see you showering their plates with chopped homegrown parsley.

If you don't have space for a window box, join a community garden.

Or ask a friend with outdoor space if you can take a bit of it to grow some tasty greens or other stuff you'd like to share.

The ultimate goal is to get your hands in the soil and wiggle them around.

Wiggle your nose around, too. Inhale and exhale slowly, through your nose, until you know what the earth smells like.

Compound that feeling with gratitude…and your spirit will grow faster than a radish.

Accumulating stuff is a privilege...and a curse. More belongings—more clothes, more electronics, more storage containers in more shapes and colors, more, more, more—doesn't bring you more happiness. It leads to physical clutter and mental muddle, and both wear down our sense of well-being, not to mention our prefrontal cortex. Take it from me, owner of way too many T-shirts, including one from the 1988 International Women's Forum in Chicago, when I introduced to the stage an unknown Chicago TV personality named Oprah Winfrey. She performed Maya Angelou's "Phenomenal Woman." If I knew then what I know now, I definitely would have had her sign the T-shirt.

Sort Yourself Out.

Remember last December 31? It was the night you popped the champagne, screamed "enough!" and resolved to do something positively healthy in the new year.

Lose thirty pounds! Go for a run three times a week! Stop after one glass of wine! (Okay, two.) Find time to meditate ten minutes a day, *no matter what!*

Proclaiming our best intentions is a piece of cake compared to sticking with them. Be honest: Have you seen a real change in yourself these last couple of months?

Don't worry. I've had cheeses last longer than many of my year-end resolutions. "Insanity," Albert Einstein told us, "is doing the same thing over and over again and expecting different results."

Dear reader, you may have tried some of my favorite action steps: Write down your goals; make them small and achievable; and keep a journal of your progress. But if you've failed time and again to make lifestyle change happen, and you want a *different* result, try doing something different, even if it strikes you as wacky.

I'm proposing that you clear the space. According to the time-honored principles of feng shui—much ridiculed, highly respected—clutter in your home and in your workspace can be a real block to change. The same is true of your mind. When you clear the space—physical and mental—magic can happen.

Christan Hummel is a pro at this. Here are a few of her best ideas, taken from her classic *Do-It-Yourself Space Clearing Kit.*

Respect your space. Energy follows thought, says Hummel. So don't bring bad energy into your home. Take off your shoes and leave them at the front door as a way to consciously let go of your concerns of the day. That was before. This is now. Now, in your home, you can shift to a more positive state. (Eastern philosophers have been teaching this for about a million years.)

Clean out bad energy. It's a subtle thing, but it just feels better to be in a personal space that is orderly and organized. Get ready to spring clean your closet, home, garage, both physically and energetically, by using essential oils like sage, smudging, or even sacred sounds. Sage? Smudging? Bells and chimes? Yep, the most effective space clearing goes way beyond Spic and Span.

Practice letting go. Make room for the new by consciously letting go of the old, on a deeply personal level. To mark the beginning of the rest of your life, perform a ritual. *Do something different.* A classic way to mark the moment is to light a candle, write down what no longer serves you—from addictions to anger—and feed it to the flame, taking care not to burn down the house.

Get rid of stuff. Your home has a circulation system, says Hummel, and when you've got too many possessions gunking it up, the energy you need to make change cannot flow. Recycle, give, or throw stuff away. Practice "emotional release work." That's when you privately honor, love, and appreciate the item (and the person who gave it to you) just before kissing it goodbye.

Another champion of sacred decluttering is Marie Kondo, the bestselling author of *The Life-Changing Magic of Tidying Up*. Her popular books and videos can be truly life-changing if you're willing to follow her KonMari method of transforming your messy spaces (and messy life) into "spaces of serenity and inspiration."

"My clients never go back to the mess," she said in one of her wildly popular sessions on YouTube. "Once you find out what objects inspire you, you find out what inspires your life."

"Tidy up in one shot," Marie Kondo advises, "as quickly, and completely, as possible." And don't go room by room. She insists you go by category, not by location—all your clothes first, all your personal mementos last, because the more you do it, the easier it gets.

"Make sure you touch each thing," says Kondo. Then listen to your body. If the item sparks joy, keep it. If it doesn't inspire you, thank it for all that it has done for you, and let it go.

ENERGY EXPRESS-O! Does That Chipped Vase Spark Joy?

"Keep only those things that speak to your heart.... By doing this you can reset your life and embark on a new lifestyle."
—Marie Kondo

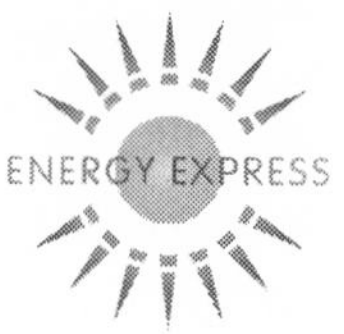

GOING DEEPER

If you think organizing your closets feels good, wait until you experience the pleasure that comes from organizing your mind.

That's the premise of a fascinating book called *Organize Your Mind, Organize Your Life: Train Your Brain to Get More Done in Less Time* by Margaret Moore, CEO of Wellcoaches, and Paul Hammerness, a Harvard Medical School psychiatrist.

Modern life is so demanding that we forget to focus. Left to our own devices, mostly digital, our prefrontal cortex is easily overwhelmed, leaving many of us feeling frenzied, distracted, and disorganized.

"It's an epidemic!" writes Moore, just like chronic multitasking. But the good news is you can train your brain to attain a higher sense of order and, along with it, a sense of calm, wisdom, positivity.

How, exactly? "Sleep well, exercise, do a mindfulness practice or choose the slow lane from time to time, even for a few minutes," writes Coach Meg, hinting at just a few of the learnable skills she and Hammerness discuss in their book.

When you organize your closet, you end up with extra space and empty hangers. When you organize your mind, you set yourself up for success in all realms.

Our bodies were meant to play and hug and have fun. That's why hunkering down at home during the pandemic created so much misery, physical and mental. That's why denying kids recess and gym in schools is such a cruel and stupid thing to do. Every body thrives when it meets the movement it loves to do. It could be softball or soccer, tango or trampoline, basketball or bocce ball. If you adore what you do, it's not work. And when you're in sync with your sport, it's not exercise. It's liberation! You are free to find joy in movement for the rest of your life.

Find Your Sport.

I've always believed there's a sport for everyone. Find it and you're home free when it comes to living an active lifestyle. Years ago, I wiggled my way into race walking, an Olympic sport unknown to me before I went to a spa retreat outside Chicago for a few days of sun and silliness with some girlfriends.

It just so happened that Olympic champion race walker Augie Hirt was giving a workshop that weekend. It changed my life. Before Augie, I was a runner—a slow, lumbering, back-of-the-pack runner. When I discovered his sport, I found mine.

As a runner, I felt like a buffalo. When I race walk, I feel like a jaguar—sleek, nimble, vibrant. I love the hip wiggle, the heel strike, the way you straighten your front leg as you stride forward, twisting your torso from side to side. Yes, it looks goofy. So what? Ever watched snowshoe baseball?

"Wear a hat," I tell friends I've taught to race walk, "and sunglasses."

Is it better than running? I think so, but you can't tell that to a runner. Race walking works your lower body *and* your upper body, and it doesn't pound your knee joints the way running does. It also works miracles on the back of your thighs where cottage cheese tends to accumulate.

I can't teach you how to race walk writing about it—it's best to learn and practice with a human guide—but I do want to tell you some things you can do to take your own walking program to a higher, more athletic level:

Shorter, faster. Any style of walking is okay when you're just getting started, but there comes a time when you need to add some zip to your step. So that means taking longer strides, right? Wrong. Take shorter, quicker ones. That's the way to go faster.

Keep your head up. This small adjustment will make a big difference. Walking with your eyes and head down is a common mistake. It strains your back and shoulder muscles, and you'll tire out quickly because it hinders efficient breathing. You are remembering to breathe, aren't you?

Move your arms. You'll be surprised how much more powerful your stride gets once you bring your arms into play. Don't hunch your shoulders or tense your arms. Allow them to swing in a relaxed and natural way, without crossing your midline in front. Keep your elbows tucked into your sides, arms bent at about a ninety-degree angle. Don't clench your fists. Keep your hands loose. Feel and move like an athlete.

Work those hips. Someday, you may want to find your own Augie Hirt-style coach and learn the official race walking technique, including one foot on the ground at all times. Meanwhile, for power walking, allow your hips to extend forward with each stride. As your right leg comes forward, so should your right hipbone, in a natural rotation. Then your left. Race walkers get a lot of speed, forward thrust, and funny looks from this exaggerated hip wiggle. It takes practice and patience, but once you get it, it's yours forever.

Engage your glutes. As you walk, practice somatics. Be aware of engaging your abdominal muscles and your glutes. Think about urging them forward under your hips, causing a bit of a pelvic tilt. Walking this way—head up, stomach and glutes engaged—is a fantastic way to help tighten and strengthen those areas that tend to get loose and flabby as we age.

Go for the roll. There's no wrong way to walk, but the right way, for maximum efficiency and power, involves walking heel-ball-toe. Focus on landing on your heel, your toes flexed to the sky, and then roll through the foot, using the big toe to give your body a powerful push forward. That way, all your leg muscles are awake and involved. Walking this way makes for a better workout, but don't overdo it. Increase your time and intensity gradually, or your shins may start to talk back to you.

So, please, dear reader, find your own sport—or grab your hat and sunglasses, and try mine. You'll find everything you need to get started at racewalking.org, and the YouTube race walking videos are good, too.

ENERGY EXPRESS-O! I'm Just Saying...

"If God had wanted people to run, he wouldn't have invented race walking."
—Rick Williams

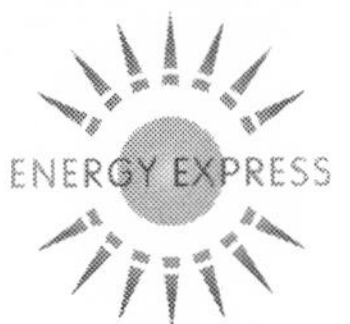

GOING DEEPER

This is a no-brainer.

Search the internet for a race walking coach or club in your town.

Yes, it's possible to learn from videos, but I still believe it's best to learn from another human being.

Your job is to find that person. If the cost is an issue, beg a friend to share a beginner's lesson with you.

Or just go with the video thing. The perfect is the enemy of the good. Start where you are with what you've got. If you want to learn, you will learn. Don't stand in your own way.

Once you get the hang of race walking, not to mention the wiggle, you may fall in love with it, and then, lucky you, you'll have found your sport. You can then practice and find it pleasurable for the rest of your life.

Don't forget your hat.

COVID disrupted our lives in countless and cruel ways, as more and more people sheltered in place and worked from home. Personally, I love not having to go into an office, but what I love even more is working at home from my standing desk. Without a doubt, it changed my life. (No one is paying me to say this. Darn.) Now I wish everyone in the world worked at a standing desk, and here's why: Chronic sitting makes you sick. Over time, it contributes to a list of diseases and ailments as long as your tibias and fibulas combined. Sitting too much blocks your energy and shortens your life. I stand amazed, and so, I hope, will you.

Stand Up for Yourself.

Sit happens. Every day, millions of Americans spend eight to fourteen hours on their behinds, sitting.

I'm talking to you.

Think about your day: You sit when you drive; watch TV; answer emails; eat breakfast, lunch, dinner, and snacks; read a book; play a video game; admire your cat. The truth is we modern Americans sit so much that it passes for totally normal behavior. We don't even think about it, do we?

Well, start thinking! Pull up your life-shortening chair, and listen to this: There are now over 10,000 studies showing that too much sitting is a terribly destructive thing to do to your health and well-being.

Rise to the truth. Your body thrives on movement, and when you make it sit for hours at a time, you create serious damage at a cellular level.

Research shows prolonged sitting significantly raises your risk of developing heart disease, obesity, diabetes, cancer, insomnia, arthritis, and osteoporosis. That's for starters. It's hard to believe chairs are still legal. If seventy is the new fifty, sitting is the new smoking.

And don't think your daily workouts will protect you. Nope. Chronic sitting is an *independent* risk factor, meaning all the risk correlations hold true no matter how much you exercise. Get it? You can exercise an hour a day and still not undo the damage that comes from too much sitting.

And that's why I want to focus not on the sitting-is-bad research (astonishing as it is), but on what you can do to sit less, micro-move more, and educate yourself about the benefits of standing:

Use a standing desk. If sitting kills, standing saves. That's why stand-up desks are quickly rising in popularity, in offices, in homes, and especially in *my* home, where I'm happily standing now, in front of my new VariDesk, a clever, affordable design in the $350 range that I've been showing off to friends like a new puppy.

Some stand-ups I researched looked too corporate and would have meant replacing my beloved old wooden desk. The VariDesk sits on top and has an easy, spring-assisted lift that takes me from sitting to standing in a couple of seconds. I love it…and I'm pretty sure it loves me.

It comes with an app for stand-up alerts, but I'm just using my own body awareness—gradually standing longer and longer until my legs tire and then sitting for thirty minutes or so before I rise again.

I found a ton of anecdotal evidence online about stand-up desks curing back pain, insomnia, fatigue, and more, and I'm not surprised. But too much standing can also create health problems (varicose veins, for instance), so stay tuned into your body, and rest in your chair when you need to.

Move more. One sure cure for too much sitting is getting up every hour and moving for ten minutes or so. Is that so hard? Apparently, yes. So do what you have to do—an app, a phone alert, a kitchen timer—to remind yourself to stand, to stretch, to do neck rolls, air squats, and other energizing movements. There's also walking to the water cooler, jumping rope, practicing your tango moves.

Mercola.com is one of many excellent resources for videos demonstrating the kind of intermittent exercises you should be doing, standing up and moving at least once every hour.

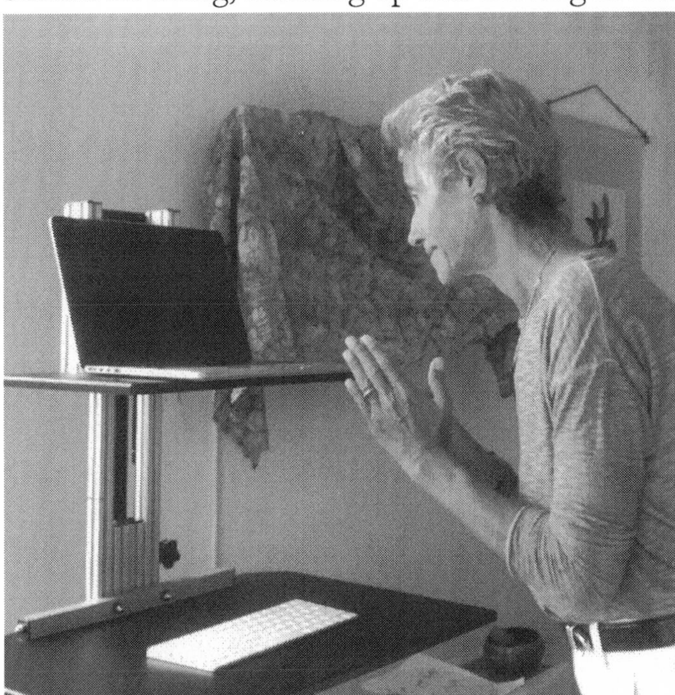

"I was able to reduce my normal twelve to fourteen hours of sitting to under one hour," Dr. Joe Mercola reports. "And I noticed one amazing thing—the back pain I've struggled with for many years simply disappeared." (Same thing happened with two of my nephews, I swear. It took a lot of nagging on my part, but it was worth it.)

Read this book. If you want to understand the solid science behind standing, read Dr. James Levine's recent book, *Get Up! Why Your Chair Is Killing You and What You Can Do About It.* He's the Mayo Clinic endocrinologist and pioneering researcher who documented the perils of too much sitting in 2000, way before it was accepted as true. And now he's a leading voice for change in the workplace, at home, and, very importantly, in schools, where prolonged sitting hurts kids and stifles creativity.

I hope you're convinced. Stand more; sit less! Now it's time for me to lower my desk and rest my…case.

ENERGY EXPRESS-O! Rise Up

"Sitting is more dangerous than smoking, kills more people than HIV and is more treacherous than parachuting. We are sitting ourselves to death."
—James Levine

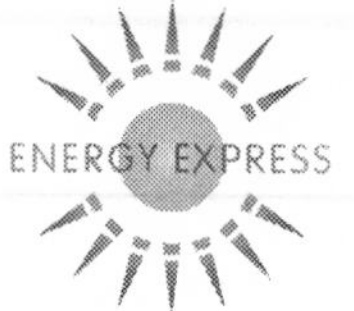

GOING DEEPER

Can you afford to replace your desk with a standing one?

My question is, can you afford not to?

Just to see what it feels like, try rigging one up at home, using books or boxes.

Ideally, you want the screen of your computer at eye level and your hands on the keyboard at a ninety-degree angle. You might want to invest in a wireless keyboard to get the proportions right.

This is important: Don't be frozen in your standing position. Unlock your knees; bounce up and down on your toes a few times; let your hips sway from side to side; pump your pelvis gently, curling and uncurling your tailbone.

Small, nourishing movements energize your body.

And when you feel tired, dear reader, please be seated. Too much standing too soon can leave you with sore legs and aching hips. As your body adjusts and gets stronger, you'll find yourself standing longer and longer.

P.S. After years of begging friends, family, and perfect strangers to please use a standing desk, I've pretty much let that go. I've trained as a coach. You can't tell another person what to do. Well, you can, but it's not going to change their behavior. People can only change themselves. I've said all I can say about the value of standing desks. But if you try one and it makes a difference, *as it has for so many people,* please rise to the occasion and spread the word.

This is going to sound weird, but I would rather learn to widen the spaces between my toes than run a marathon. It's true. Nothing against marathons, but one of the greatest discoveries I've made on the path to personal well-being involves the value of somatic awareness, the making of teeny-tiny movements inside your body, guided by your mind's eye, empowered by your breath. Expand the butterfly wings of your back. Float your diaphragm. Lift energy from the arches of your feet to the crown of your head. Is this even possible? Yes! Somatic movements engage the subtle energies and awaken your whole body. The practice looks passive—you can do it lying on your back—but in fact, it's wildly powerful. Don't turn me in to the AMA, but I've successfully used somatic movements to relieve a painful shoulder, unblock a jammed knee, and otherwise infuriate many M.D. pals of mine who have no idea what I'm talking about.

Start Very Small.

When we humans imagine ourselves "exercising," we focus on playing sports, working out in the gym, going for a walk. Yes! All great ways to boost your energy and give your body the juiciness and joy it deserves.

But please don't limit your exercise routine to these big-picture pursuits. There is the outer game—played out on soccer fields, tennis courts, treadmills—but there's an inner game, too, going on inside every interconnected nerve, cell, muscle, fascia, and bone of your body.

And if you're not making *that* connection, you're missing out on a wonderful, even magical, opportunity to boost your strength and improve your well-being.

Sense your sacrum. Let's focus on the sacrum to begin to shift your thinking. Do you know precisely where yours is? You should. Your sacrum—the Greek word for "sacred bone," where the ancients believed the soul resides—is holy ground when it comes to the health of your lower back, your legs, your knees, your everything.

It is centrally located at the base of your spine, and if it's not stable, strong, and in balance, it can pinch, bite, and break you, in the form of back pain, leg pain, numbness, tingling, and worse.

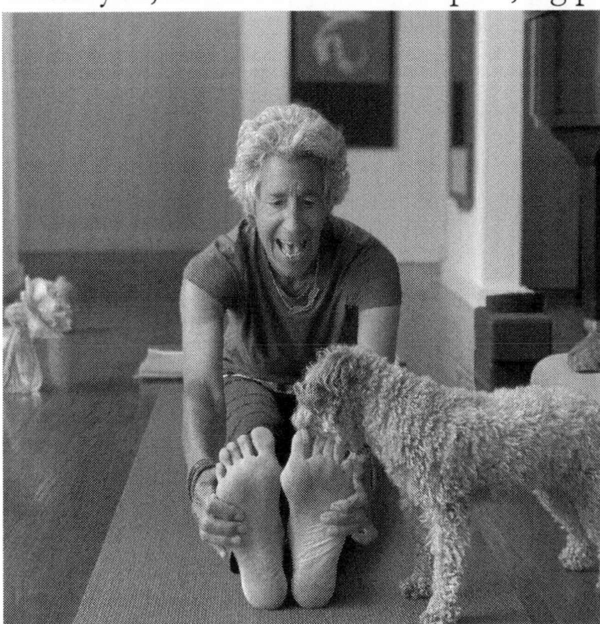

The inner game begins as you connect to your skeletal-muscular self, using an anatomy book for guidance or learning from an evolved teacher or engaging with the detailed images at www.innerbody.com, where you can pilot through the body using 3-D rotating images.

So, zoom in on the sacrum, the large triangular-shaped vertebrae that joins up with your hipbones to form your pelvis.

Admire the architecture, front and back, right and left side. Notice how it sits between the two pelvic crests (called the ilium). Now find your own sacrum. Frame your two hands around it. I like to relax my thumbs onto my pelvic bone and flip my fingers around so they are pointed toward my spine, resting on both sides of the sacrum. Hello, sacrum. How ya hanging?

Find your SI joint. Between the sacrum and the ilium is

the notorious sacroiliac joint, or SI joint. The SI joint stabilizes your pelvis and lower spine whenever you do any kind of movement. If you want a sustainable career as a walker, runner, tennis player, square dancer, or pole dancer, you want to nourish and protect a strong, flexible SI joint.

And here's another ain't-nature-grand fact. When you're young, your sacrum starts out as five individual bones, or vertebrae. During late adolescence, the five vertebrae begin to merge, and by the time most of us are thirty years old, our sacrum has formed into one single bone, roughly the size of your hand.

Your sacrum is a very strong bone, because it has to be. Besides protecting all the spinal nerves of the lower back, and the entire female reproductive system, the sacrum supports the weight of the upper body as it spreads across the pelvis into the legs. It also locks the hipbones together on the back and supports the base of the spinal column as it interacts with the pelvis. The bone itself has a spongy interior, and it appreciates nourishing fluids.

A happy sacrum is a balanced sacrum. Once you focus on the architecture of your sacrum—complex, connected—you'll understand why having a sense of it makes sense.

How does your sacrum feel when you bend forward from the waist slowly? Or arch your back? Is there tightness? Imbalance? Are there twinges?

Self-care clicks in when you sense and listen to your body, to the clues it's giving you about how it feels, how not to hurt it, what it needs.

And what it needs in the sacral region is stability, strength, and enough juice to keep the nerves that pass through the sacrum moist and happy.

Which brings us back to exercise, and the science of

going small, with somatics training, physical therapy, yoga, Qigong, the Alexander Technique, Pilates, Feldenkrais, and more.

Even the best doctors were flat-out wrong when they used to tell people with lower-back pain to go to bed and rest their back until it got better. The opposite is true. Now doctors will tell you that it's slow, subtle, gentle exercise that helps ease the pain and promotes healing.

They know better now, and so do you. Find a path to somatics training. Start small; finish healthy.

ENERGY EXPRESS-O! The Body Is Amazing

"This new mode of functioning awakens us to the amazing self-sensing, self-organizing, and self-renewing system that we are."
—Risa F. Kaparo

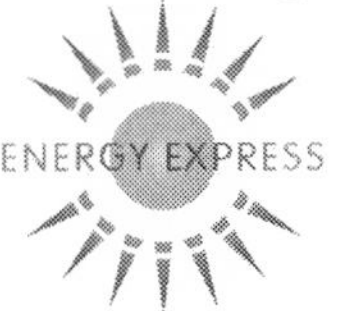

GOING DEEPER

There's nothing like reading a good book.

Unless it's reading three very good books, all about somatics. If you don't educate yourself, how will it happen?

One I find especially informative is by my friend Tias Little, a master yoga teacher. It's called *Yoga of the Subtle Body: A Guide to the Physical and Energetic Anatomy of Yoga*, an elegant and dense book steeped in poetry and metaphor, not to mention anatomy, physiology, and neuroscience.

Somatics: Reawakening the Mind's Control of Movement, Flexibility, and Health is the groundbreaking classic by Thomas Hanna. Motor sensory awareness is his thing, and his five-minute daily program is one that can help almost anyone "maintain the pleasures of a supple, healthy body."

Another inspiring and innovative work is *Awakening Somatic Intelligence: The Art and Practice of Embodied Mindfulness* by psychotherapist Risa Kaparo, Ph.D. It incorporates mindfulness, visualization, breathing exercises, postures, and stretches into one big life-changing whole.

Pick one. Read it. Then put it into practice. Discover why making the mind-body connection is such a useful tool to have in your healthy lifestyle toolbox, unlike, let's say, chemical-laden sunscreens.

Bodybuilders use visualization to target, grow, and relax their muscles in very precise ways. So do students of yin yoga, a kind of therapeutic yoga that is very helpful for recuperating after an injury. "You don't use your body to find the pose," it teaches. "You use the pose to find your body." Yes! When you link to your body, slowly, through your breath, you can go deeper into your pose, your sport, your everyday experience of life. Lengthen your tailbone. Open the wings of your lungs. Balance your pelvis so it feels like a swing on a swing set. Is your imagination really making a difference? Is your tailbone actually longer? I promise you, it doesn't matter.

Think in Pictures.

The stress and uncertainty of COVID battered our bodies day after day, fear after fear. The tight shoulders, the sore neck, the nagging ache that seizes your lower back and locks it in pain. We've all been there, and waiting for life to return to whatever normal looks like only makes the suffering worse.

Which is why I want to introduce you to yin yoga. It's unique characteristic is long, three-to-five-minute holds, combined with subtle pumps, slow stretches, conscious breathing, and eye-opening visualizations. You begin to think in pictures, something world-champion skiers, swimmers, and basketball players do, too.

This ancient practice is the pause that truly refreshes. It's about as far from situps and pullups as kite surfing is from floating in a pool with a mojito in your hand.

And here's the part you must believe: Yin yoga is accessible to all, even if you don't know a tree pose from a tree frog.

I took two yin yoga classes last week—in my family, we call this research—and at some point, as my constricted chest opened and I imagined warm honey pouring out of my heart, I had a revelation. This little-known form of yoga—this blissful experience of letting go and creating flow—is a wonderful way to become more flexible, less stuck, physically and mentally. And it's so easy. If only people knew!

So, let's begin. In all of yoga, you start where you are, but with yin yoga, it's especially true. It's a class in deep release and relaxation, what some teachers call restorative yoga. But yin yoga has its own special twist.

For one thing, it moves very slowly. In an hour or so, you might only get to five or six different postures. Be grateful for these long holds. They're a wonderful way, perhaps the only way, to release the bands of connective tissue that only get tighter and more restrictive as we age, as we sit, as we move too quickly through life. (You talking to me?)

Most exercise we do—running, biking, dynamic forms of yoga like ashtanga—is considered yang. In simplest Taoist terms, yang is the expansion force; yin is the contracting force. Yang exercise works on muscle through rhythm and repetition but does zilch for your connective tissue, your fascia. And that's what we humans want to access to have a more fluid and healthy body.

In a yin yoga class, you're given instruction, and permission, to mindfully explore and expand the tight connective tissue. Your breath is clearing the way—mentally and physically—for a healing flow of energy into and surrounding your hips, your knees, your spine.

The trick to loving your yin yoga class is learning what to do with yourself once you've eased into your posture. Five minutes can be boring, or it can be a journey of exploration, an active experience of tuning in, letting go.

First, you might give in to the desire to look around the room to see who's holding their toes and who can't even see them. When you decide to keep your eyes on your own mat, you've discovered something valuable: Yoga is not a competitive sport. Someone is *always* more supple than you are. So what?

Second, instead of those sideways glances, direct your focus inside. Visualize the deepest part of your structure relaxing, expanding, pulsing. Think in pictures. Once your mind sees it, your body will follow. Be patient. When you experience your edge, back off. You'll still make progress, but you won't wind up with an injury.

Third, play with your breath. It's not a religious belief. It's a way of connecting your body to your mind. Make the effort, and you'll feel the effect. When you go with the flow, your breath helps unblock and release, opening up and juicing up what is known in yoga as the subtle body.

There's nothing subtle about the benefits of this kind of practice. So here are some highlights from a life-changing workshop I did with yin yoga master Paul Grilley some years ago in Chicago. He's been teaching since 1980, and his website is a wonderful resource for yin yoga information and study, including his revealing collection of bone photos.

Yin yoga stills, and then restarts, the flow of energy. Grilley teaches you that your connective tissue isn't just some inert gristle that keeps your knees in place and your back from going out.

Your connective tissue is a river of life-giving energy that flows through your entire body. It follows the meridian pathways described in the ancient texts on acupuncture, a flow of energy (also known as "chi") that can reach and nourish every cell and organ in your body.

Accept what is. Grilley began our workshop by pulling thighbones and pelvises out of a canvas bag and laying them on the floor. Talk about an attention-getter. Structural limitation is real, says Grilley, pointing to all the shapes and sizes laid before us.

As an anatomy expert, he wants you to understand that the unique angle and shape of your bones determines what you can do in yoga, no matter how many hours you spend willing your head to touch your toes.

"Your anatomy is yours! Your femur is different from the person's next to you! All your good intentions and instruction—relax and let it open!—can't push you past your compression point."

Translation? You may never do the splits or sit in full lotus, no matter how hard you push. That's okay, says Grilley. Focus your attention within the pose, not on how it looks, but how it feels.

"Yoga isn't about imitating a posture; it's about unblocking energy, moving your chi."

Chi whiz.

ENERGY EXPRESS-O! Why We Practice

"Yoga is the perfect opportunity to be curious about who you are."
—Jason Crandell

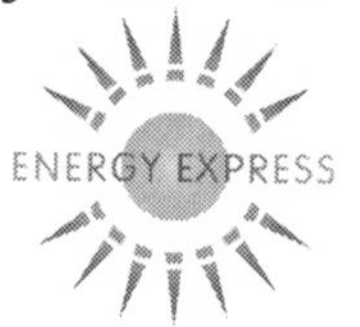

GOING DEEPER

Yin yoga involves the doing of specific postures, or asanas, but I hope you realize that the practice of yoga goes way beyond the practice of doing postures.

Yoga is a multilayered philosophy of living and breathing and being. It calls on you to be kind and loving to yourself and others, even when they piss you off.

Yoga can also help you deal with negative emotions, like anger, depression, anxiety. So can running, photography, and gardening, but I keep coming back to the yoga path because it's so well-documented, so filled with unexpected moments of clarity.

When COVID hit, and gyms shut down, lots of people saw this as an opportunity to do more yoga, at home, free and convenient, with a minimum of props and a maximum of privacy.

Sounds good…but. What many people discover is that most yoga classes online move too quickly to follow along safely. If you already know the poses and how to do them properly, in alignment, never pushing into the pain, great. If you are new to yoga and lurching mindlessly from pose to pose, online classes or videos may lead to injuries.

Yin yoga is the exception because it moves slowly and deliberately. The best way to go deeper is to find an experienced, inspired yin yoga teacher and go to at least one class, just to see if you want to stick with it.

Reread this chapter before every session.

If you find yin yoga boring, explore that sensation without giving it a name. Just witness yourself being bored.

Then shift your focus to your breathing, in and out of your nose, slowly, engaging your diaphragm while you search for hot spots. What's that feeling in your hamstring? How's your low back reacting? What little adjustment might create more space in your shoulder joint?

When you get that mind-body conversation going, you'll notice that your boredom is transformed into something else. You don't have to give that a name either. Just notice it.

Ideally, you'll entice a friend to experience some yin yoga classes with you. It's fun to have someone to talk to, to listen to, when class is over.

Misery loves company, but so does bliss.

The global pandemic undercut and overwhelmed our sense of happiness. The deaths, the despair, the dreams delayed or destroyed shook us to our core. Recovery will take the time it takes. While the uncertainty of what's ahead continues to unfold, here's one thing I know for sure: Our personal well-being ultimately depends on our own choices: how active, compassionate, and mindful we are; how much sleep we get; what we eat and drink; how much love and grace we have in our life; and, yes, how happy we want to be.

Choose to Be Happy.

We are living in a world turned upside down by a virus of unknown origin. Personal well-being is under assault like never before. What will happen? When will we return to normal, knowing that normal is past tense and never coming back? What can a healthy lifestyle expert offer to inspire her readers who are suffering in ways they never expected?

Unconditional Happiness! It's one of my favorite classes at the University of Well-Being, Ballet, and Refrigeration because it's so controversial, so fascinating to consider, so essential if we are to remain strong and clear and move on with our lives in a way that promotes healing, defeats depression, and uncurls our toes.

Unconditional Happiness is the practice of choosing to be happy, no matter what. No matter who has died or lied, no matter the state of our divided nation, you can lift your spirit and boost your health by answering this one question: "Do I want to be happy, or do I not want to be happy?"

Michael Singer, an expert in Unconditional Happiness, calls it a simple question. But for most of us, it's impossibly complex. How can you be happy when you lose your business, your kids are miserable, and your health care system screws up so badly you're left to fend for yourself, more or less, with the vaccine or without?

"Once you decide you want to be unconditionally happy, something inevitably will happen that challenges you," Singer explains in his New York Times bestseller, *The Untethered Soul.*

Accept your life as it unfolds, Singer teaches. Don't let what happens make you miserable. If your answer to the "Do I want to be happy?" question is yes, then you have to let go of all conditions that arise. "You have to mean it regardless of what happens."

Even when what happens is something as catastrophic as the global pandemic. I told you it was controversial.

"When everything is going well, it's easy to be happy," writes Singer, who went from a penniless yogi to the founding CEO of a billion-dollar public company. "But the moment something difficult happens, it's not so easy."

"The question is not whether they will happen," Singer writes. "Things are going to happen. The real question is whether you want to be happy regardless of what happens. The purpose of your life is to enjoy and learn from your experiences. You were not put on Earth to suffer. You're not helping anybody by being miserable."

You can and should be vigilant, concerned, aware, involved in whatever distressing situation comes your way, Singer explains, but you can't let it get in the way of your commitment to be happy. Well, you can, but that's not the path to personal well-being.

"Committing yourself to unconditional happiness will teach you every single thing there is to learn about yourself, about others, about the nature of life," says Singer. "You will learn all about your mind, your heart, and your will. But you have to mean it when you say that you'll be happy for the rest of your life. Every time a part of you begins to get unhappy, let it go."

Easier said than done, it's true, especially when COVID hit so many, so hard, but here's something else that's true.

"Regardless of your philosophical beliefs, the fact remains that you were born and you are going to die. During the time in between, you get to choose whether or not you want to enjoy the experience.

"Events don't determine whether or not you're going to be happy. They're just events. You determine whether or not you're going to be happy. You can be happy just to be alive. You can be happy having all these things happen to you, and then be happy to die."

Singer sets a high bar, especially for those who prefer going to a bar when something awful happens.

"If you want to be happy, you have to let go of the part of you that wants to create melodrama. This is the part that thinks there's a reason not to be happy. You have to transcend the personal, and as you do, you will naturally awaken to the higher aspects of your being."

That's when that overwhelming feeling of well-being kicks in, because you've made that strong choice.

"No matter what happens, just enjoy the life that comes to you," Singer says.

No matter what.

ENERGY EXPRESS-O! Hungry for a Laugh?

"I'm not crazy about reality, but it's still the only place to get a decent meal."
—Groucho Marx

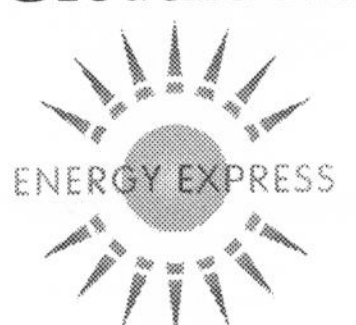

GOING DEEPER

Jack Kornfield—a bestselling author and world class meditation teacher—is someone to turn to when the sky turns dark and fear overcomes you and all you can see are terrifying times ahead.

"When times are uncertain, difficult, fearful, full of change," Jack writes, "they become the perfect place to deepen the practice of awakening."

Are you up for an awakening? Maybe you already had one during the worst times of COVID. Maybe you realized that having dinner with your family made you happier than staying late at the office. Maybe you woke up to the need to acquire less, relate better, add more plant-based protein to your dinner plate.

Becoming awake and aware is at the heart of personal well-being, and so are these suggestions from Susan Piver, founder of the Open Heart Project:

Be generous. When we are afraid, we feel powerless. However, generosity is a gesture of power. So, if you are feeling numb, aggressive, fearful, reach out and help someone else who is struggling. It's good for others, Piver says, and it's a very good thing to do for ourselves.

Remember that nothing is ever, ever as good as you hope or as bad as you fear. Take it one day at a time, Piver says. One day, one thought, one moment at a time. Meditation teaches you how to meet your experience on the spot, fully and courageously. Practice every day for maximum benefit, even if it's just for five or ten minutes.

Elect yourself president. "Your life—your home, family, friends, workplace, body, abilities—are your kingdom," writes Piver. You're the ruler in charge. What can you do for your world? Who or what needs your attention? Now is the time for you to remove every obstacle that stands in the way of doing your true work in the world. Start where you are; do your best; accept the outcome without blaming anyone, including yourself.

Express your love for your brothers and sisters. Piver isn't suggesting that we get all snuggly with the hatemongers, the racists, the antisemites, but she asks us to acknowledge we are all Americans. This is our country. United we stand, divided we get very, very nervous. Seeking to excise fifty percent of our brothers and sisters from our hearts and minds is not the higher path, and it extends suffering.

Feel what you feel. Don't pretend you aren't scared, sad, angry, and shocked, if you are. That's not a problem. What is a problem is to ignore what you feel and take it out on others by vilifying them. Terrible people must be held accountable for terrible things. But grasping at aggression keeps us from seeing clearly the best course of action.

And what is the best course of action? Awaken.

When I was growing up—taught by my softball-loving dad to catch and throw "like a boy"—girls were never encouraged to work with weights. "It's not feminine." "You'll bulk up." Crapola of all sorts. Strength training was for the guys, while the girls at South Shore High School earned gym credits for keeping their shoes chalked white and their hideous green gym suits starched and ironed. That was then. This is now. Now is about a million times better.

Play to Your Strength.

You can run a 10K every weekend, or hike, bike, and play tennis from morning to night, and *still* the most efficient way to build muscle and overall body strength is targeted strength training.

There are many good reasons for strength training beyond looking good in a swimsuit. Strong bodies are linked to strong minds. Strength training builds confidence, muscle, and healthy tissue. It's also good for stable joints, injury prevention, and weight loss. And yet—slugs that we are—fewer than twenty-five percent of Americans over the age of forty-five work with weights on a regular basis. A whole lot fewer, I'm guessing.

Blame it on our sedentary lifestyles. The heaviest thing most of us lift is our laptop. Nothing we do requires us to raise our arms over our heads. Everyday chores may work the front body, but what about the back body, the side body, the subtle body inside your own body that benefits from a balanced program that builds muscle from top to bottom, back to front, side to side?

So, for all those reasons and a superset more, here are eight strength-training truths to consider—as you decide how and when you'll either get started or jump back in:

There's no age limit. Little kids have to wait until their bodies and bones are strong enough to take the stresses of weight training, but the rest of us can start where we are and can expect to see big improvements over time. The body is magnificent that way. People in their nineties are pumping iron and getting stronger, and so will you, once you understand the basics.

Technique is everything. This is a weighty matter, because if you don't learn to lift consciously, with awareness of your breath, posture, core, and limitations, you can strain a muscle or tear a tendon. Find an evolved teacher/trainer, or teach yourself from books or online videos.

Lift heavier weights. You won't get stronger lifting the same five- or ten-pound weight day after day, rep after rep. For your muscles to grow stronger, you need to challenge them—gradually, over time—with heavier weights. The "right" amount of weight will always vary, but this principle remains the same: You should be able to do ten or so reps with perfect form, with the last two being a real struggle.

Machines versus free weights. Both will build strength. Using machines in a gym usually comes with a price tag. Free weights speak for themselves, anytime, anywhere. Machines have a limited range of motion; free weights have infinite possibilities. *Both* can work if you work, intensely, consistently, thoughtfully, with proper attention paid to form and breathing. Body-weight exercises—squats, pushups, lunges—should also be part of your routine, which is why it's smart to consult with someone knowledgeable when you're first starting.

(Yoga, as you know, uses your own body weight to get you strong and supple, sculpting your muscles into pleasing shapes while building tremendous strength in your core, your arms and legs, your hips and shoulders. But in this chapter, I want to shine a light on weightlifting the traditional way, just to show you how well-rounded I can be.)

Expect soreness. It's called DOMS—delayed onset muscle soreness—and it's what you can expect after a good workout. Pain is different. "No pain, no gain" is no way to approach a sustainable strength-training practice. If your trainer thinks otherwise, find one with a heftier brain.

Know your body. Spend some time looking at anatomical drawings so you'll know your kidney from your colon, your patella from your pubic bone. Developing better body awareness will help you create and execute a balanced workout: front to back, side to side, pushing and pulling, expanding and contracting, pumping just enough to experience the pleasure.

Be efficient. A twenty-minute workout can be just as good as a forty-minute workout, if you know what you're doing and why. Compound movements, for example—a bicep curl combined with a lunge—will give you twice the benefit in half the time. So will super-slow lifting and high-intensity interval training. Some people love super-slow lifting; others would rather be eaten by a shark.

Again, study up and experiment until you find a routine that sparks joy. If you manage to do it two or three times a week, over time, your body will change in remarkable ways, unless you celebrate every workout with two granola bars and three beers.

Use it or lose it. It's an inconvenient truth that as we age, we lose muscle and grow weak UNLESS we make the effort to stay strong, flexible, agile, and juiced. It's about working with what you've got for as long as you've got, and being grateful in between.

ENERGY EXPRESS-O: The Reason We Train

"It is never too late to be what you might have been."
—George Eliot

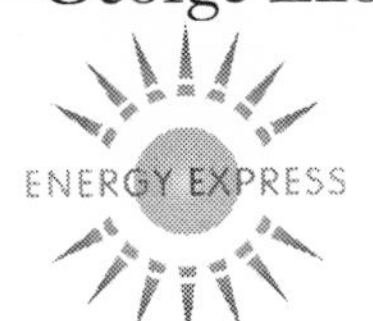

GOING DEEPER

If you decide to lift weights, I urge you to buy some time with a trainer who can teach you proper breathing and how to find pleasure in the process of building strength.

These are learnable skills, and when you feel ready, you can drop the coaching and continue on your own.

But if you start off doing it wrong—holding your breath, jerking the weights, moving too quickly—you can create injuries, miseries, and doctors' bills.

Another good idea for going deeper is to find a good motivational book on strength training, one that focuses less on technique and more on the seductive nature of bodybuilding.

Rick Newcombe's *The Magic of Lifting Weights* is that kind of book.

(Full disclosure: Rick is the founder of Creators, the publisher of this book you're reading. He's been a body builder for more than fifty years. His arms are the size of Duke footballs, and if you ever wanted someone to sell you on the life-enriching joys of pumping iron, Rick's your guy.)

Here's one of his best tips.

"My trainer says the best workout is twenty minutes of stretching, twenty minutes of cardio, and twenty minutes of weights," Rick's daughter, Sara, told him one day. "You've been working out your whole life, Dad. Do you think he's right?"

Rick thought for a while. The number one best workout to build your strength? Sounds like a loaded question to me.

"The majority of people want to exercise but don't stick with it. Of the ones who do, what they have in common is that they enjoy their workouts." Rick told her. "The more I think about it, Sara, I would say the best workout is the one you like enough to keep doing it."

Pumping gold.

Summer

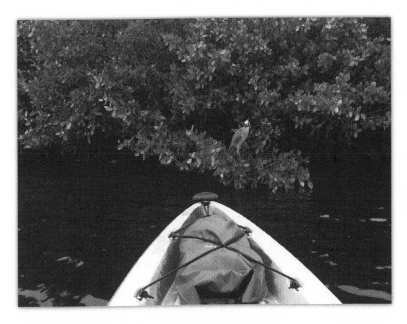

Robinson Preserve, Florida

"Summer afternoon—summer afternoon; to me, those have always been the two most beautiful words in the English language."
—Henry James

"There's this magical sense of possibility that stretches like a bridge between June and August. A sense that anything can happen."
—Aimee Friedman

"Some of the best memories are made in flip flops."
— Kellie Elmore

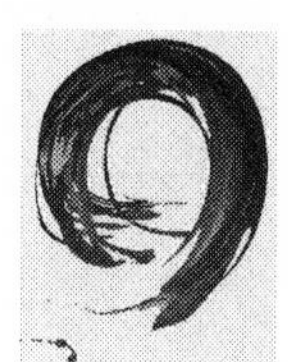

I plan to grow up to be a magnificent elder. Look at the old lady in the punky haircut, they'll say, loved and loving at ninety-three, still hiking, still laughing, still dancing till dawn (okay, midnight). A long life is part luck, part grace, and—what else? I'd always wondered. And then I discovered the Blue Zones. The mystery of exceptional aging is no mystery at all. There are guidelines to be followed, insights to be shared, rules we can respect. One of my favorites involves waking up every morning with a passion and a purpose that gives your life meaning. When that ends, so will you.

Live Long, Die Happy.

This is the time of year I live, play, and work on a tiny, remote Greek island with no airport and fewer than three thousand residents, not including the goats.

It's a beautiful, magical, revelatory place. Be happy for me. A generous spirit is a sign that your healthy lifestyle training is paying off.

Of course, I take the World Wide Web with me, so anxiety-producing news is never far away. And neither is the island of Ikaria, one of the world-famous Blue Zones, seven well-studied communities where surprisingly large numbers of people live into their nineties and beyond and are vigorous, healthy, and relatively happy right to the end.

I can see Ikaria from my terrace, high above the Aegean, sipping a glass of cold retsina, chipping away at a chunk of freshly made feta cheese with wild oregano on top. It's a form of research. It inspires me to ask this age-old question:

Why do some people live so much longer than others?

Genetics play only a small part in longevity, twenty percent or less. Much more important are your personal lifestyle choices: what you eat and drink; the amount of physical activity you do; the time you spend with family and friends; how you handle tension, trauma, the ticking of the clock.

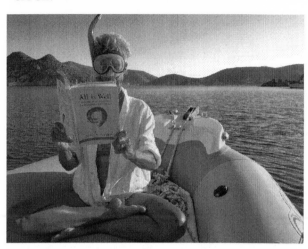

Ikaria—twenty-five miles long, five miles wide, with healing hot springs that have made it a tourist attraction since 600 B.C.—has been studied up one mountainside and down the other. Blue Zone researchers want to determine what keeps Ikarians living so long, so well, with so little heart disease and diabetes, and virtually no dementia.

Let me repeat that last part before I forget: In Ikaria, dementia is practically unknown. In the U.S., dementia is rampant, costly, and incredibly scary.

In the U.S., only one in nine baby boomers will live to the age of ninety, according to Dan Buettner, head of the Blue Zone movement. On Ikaria, one in three live to ninety and beyond.

Amazing. What do they know that we've forgotten?

You can find the answers in great detail at BlueZones.com. However, here's my summary, after spending some sweet days walking and talking my way around Ikaria. I hope you're not too busy to read it:

Take your time. To live longer, slow down. On Ikaria, wristwatches are as useless as speed bumps. Ikarians are famous for moving at their own pace, working when they want to work, chilling when they want to chill. I learned that

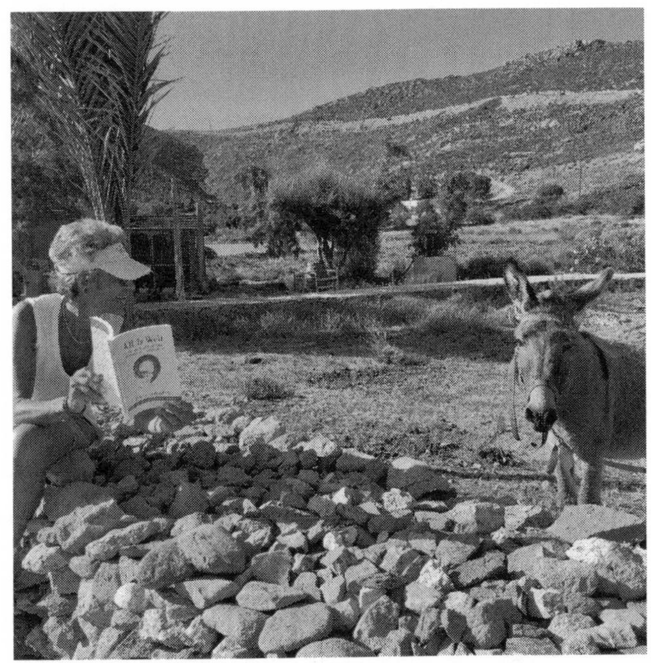

on my first visit there, having lunch with friends at a wonderful little taverna in the port of Agios Kirikos. We all ordered Greek salads. Some of us are still waiting.

Eat your greens. Over 150 kinds of wild greens grow all over the island, and Ikarians enjoy them in a variety of unusual salads and pies. It takes just the slightest bit of courage to stick your fork in. The island greens are a super source of antioxidants and are eaten, like almost everything else, with a splash of olive oil.

Drink herbal tea. Ikarians drink endless cups of tea made from wild mint, chamomile, and other local herbs high in compounds that significantly lower blood pressure and decrease their risk of heart disease and dementia.

Take a nap. Ikarians take daily naps (about thirty minutes) at least five times a week. Blue Zone researchers calculate this lowers their risk of heart attacks by thirty-five percent! In a few of the mountain villages, they sleep by day and work and play through the night. Why? Because they want to.

(FYI: "Based on interviews," says Blue Zones expert Dan

Buettner, "we have reason to believe that most Ikarians over ninety are sexually active.")

Keep moving. Many Ikarians live in mountain villages that require vigorous walking. They keep terraced gardens, tend to animals, and get lots of exercise every day without thinking about it.

Connect to community. Ikarians maintain strong social ties to their families, neighbors, and villages. They wake up feeling they have a purpose in life, whether it's tending to the great-grandchildren or feeding their chickens. They take time every day to meet face to face with friends, sipping ouzo, shooting the breeze.

Eat the Ikarian way. Ikarians thrive on local fresh food, all of it organic and unprocessed. They avoid most dairy but consume gallons of goat's milk as yogurt or cheese. Their version of the gold-standard Mediterranean diet is high in fruits and vegetables, beans, whole grains, potatoes, and olive oil. They drink a glass or two of local wine—absent nitrates and pesticides. (Some folks think it tastes like rotted leaf mulch; I like it. It could be a case of mind over matter.) And they benefit hugely from daily doses of their local honey, a thick, amber-colored concoction rich in antibacterial and anti-inflammatory compounds.

Each of these Blue Zone guidelines could be a book. There is so much more to say, to do, to be. Maybe another time. You're free to go now. Time for a life-extending nap.

ENERGY EXPRESS-O! The Blue Pearl Zone

"In the end, all that really matters is the state of your heart."
—Swami Chidvilasananda

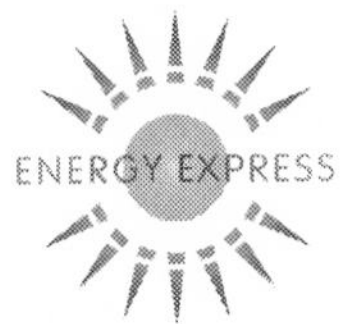

GOING DEEPER

Choose one of the Blue Zone rules, and plug it into your own life, no matter where you live or how old you are.

More time with friends? Guilt-free naps? More walks, less worry?

If you can't decide, try this one: Give yourself four olive-filled weeks on the Mediterranean diet. I choke on the word "diet," but in this case, it's come to mean a lifestyle choice, a super healthy way of eating that has nothing to do with denial and deprivation and everything to do with consuming real food, in moderate amounts, with a focus on fruits and vegetables, olive oil, whole grains, lean meats, and fresh fish. There are many variations, but the core principles are the same, including a modest pour of red wine and slowing down enough to savor every sip, every bite.

The Med diet isn't for everyone. But in study after study, it keeps coming out on top as a way of eating that is good for all sorts of Westerners who want more energy, less bloat, and, over time, a comfortable, sustainable weight.

It's not about being thin. It's about eating real food, with real taste, and real advantages to your health and wellness.

If you come to love the Med diet, and it becomes part of your lifestyle, bravo.

Next step? A week on Ikaria, possibly two.

P.S. Creators, the publisher of this book, is based in Hermosa Beach, California—a Blue Zone community.

I grew up loving sports. I wish I could say the same for French or Algebra. Early on, my folks stepped up to the plate and made sure my sister and I knew how to ride a bike, hit a ball, swim, bowl, roller skate, jump rope, ride a horse, and play tennis, golf, even horse shoes. It never mattered that we weren't the best. The message was: Have fun; learn something new; be a team player; don't break anything. I created "Energy Express," the Emmy-winning syndicated TV series about sports, fitness, and adventure, to inspire millions of kids to grow up loving to be active. It all begins when you're little.

Raise an Active Kid.

"Hit the ball! You're not concentrating!"

"Your baby brother could have caught that!"

"Run! Faster! You're not even trying!"

Lots of parents don't know how to behave when they watch their kid play sports. They're loud and obnoxious and super-critical. So, how should they act? Differently.

Here are some vital parenting rules to help you lead your child into a life of active play so they don't give up and drop out of sports before they've had a chance to find the one they love—as long as it's not football:

Be positive. If you can't say something nice during a game, say nothing at all. Or stay home. You're the parent, not the coach. Your job is to be supportive, encouraging, unconditionally loving. Keep your comments positive. Let go of the negative. Give your kid credit for showing up, for working well with her teammates, for being a good sport. These qualities are a thousand times more important to your kid's future well-being than the final score of the game.

Focus on fun. If you want your kids to relax and enjoy sports, you have to relax and enjoy watching. If you get upset and unruly, so will they. All the experts agree: The quickest way to kill a kid's interest in sports is to overemphasize winning. It's a game! The real victory is for your kid to feel comfortable and happy chasing a tennis ball or swinging a bat. Kids who are made to feel unworthy on the field take that insecurity into adulthood. It's not pretty.

Praise the effort in spite of the outcome. If your kid's team wins the game, bravo. But if your youngster is on the losing side, you need to offer empathy, not criticism. Recognize the loss, but don't dwell on it. The teachable moment is not about the value of winning but the value of resiliency. If you can develop that nothing-can-defeat-me spirit as a kid, being an adult gets a whole lot easier. Instead of dwelling on the loss, shift your kid's focus to something positive. Ask: What was the best part of the game?

Be available. Your behavior on game day is important, but a winning attitude at home counts, too. Do less talking and a lot more listening to your kid's experience. Don't judge. And don't box them in to playing soccer just because you grew up with posters of Pelé in your room. Go join an adult soccer league and let your kids figure out what they love. Irish dancing? Trampoline? Cave diving? (God forbid.)

Stay above the fray. Sometimes, fights erupt at a game, in the stands, on the field. Stay out of it. Don't abuse the refs or boo the other team. Stay cool; take a few calming breaths; and eat some apple slices till the argument blows over. It's also unwise to be critical of a coach in front of your kids. If you've got a question or complaint, take it up privately.

Keep your eye on the prize. Research shows that most kids play sports to have fun, improve their skills, and socialize with their friends. Winning isn't as big a deal to kids as it is to adults.

A much bigger deal is having your daughter or son feel good after the game. Fake praise won't do it. Kids are smarter than that.

If you parent with positive feedback and compassion when it comes to sports, your kid is much more likely to grow up enjoying an active, healthy lifestyle.

And that's the real goal, isn't it?

ENERGY EXPRESS-O! Try This on Your Kid

"We didn't lose the game. We just ran out of time."
—Vince Lombardi

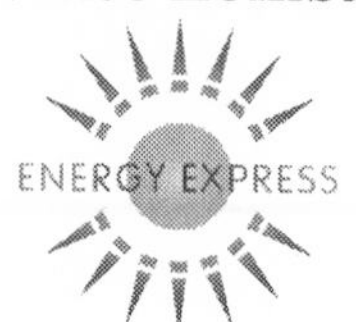

GOING DEEPER

Kids just want to play and learn stuff and have fun and see their friends, COVID or no COVID.

That's why the school shutdowns were such an existential nightmare. The extent of the damage done is still unfolding, but we know our kids took a hit, mentally and physically. Their parents may never recover.

What to do? Stop agonizing over what you can't control, and take action in a way that brings joy. Plan a special outdoor play date with your own child, or one in your life.

Here's the twist: Pick a sport neither of you has ever tried.

Cross-country skiing? Bird-watching? Ping-pong?

Reread my "Raise An Active Kid" essay the night before you head out.

And again in the morning.

Remember that your goal, your objective, is to have a day

of fun together.

Don't keep score. Leave your devices in the car. Keep laughing; keep smiling.

Win or lose, the goal is for both of you to end the day feeling like champions.

I know I'm a pain when it comes to promoting self-care. Someone shut me up. No one likes a nag. And yet, I can't resist: If our mutually horrifying experience of COVID-19 taught us anything, it's this: When push comes to pandemic, your well-being is your responsibility. The government can't save you. The best doctors can't save you. Yes, we need skilled and compassionate health care workers to help us through. And yes, there are miracle drugs and therapies that save lives. But in the end, it's your life, made up of your personal choices, big and small, from how you deal with stress to what you eat to how you breathe. You are remembering to nasal breathe, aren't you?

Wake Up to Awareness.

Aches and pains are part of life. You wake up one morning, and your back is tight, your shoulder is sore, your neck is jammed between two stone pillars. We usually accept these limitations and move on the best we can, with or without an aspirin.

But here's the good news. Many of the aches and pains we live with or take painkillers for are caused by muscular imbalance. And muscular imbalance is often curable. *By us*, no prescription, no surgery, required.

Muscle imbalance is what happens when you use one set of muscles too much and the opposing muscles a lot less.

It happens to everyone. You know what else happens? Costly visits to doctors. The tight, overused muscles—over time—become inflamed and irritated. The underused muscles weaken and become vulnerable.

Once you realize how locked in you and your body are to repetitive patterns, you can begin to reprogram. It takes focused body awareness—also known as somatics training—which is probably why attention rhymes with prevention.

To prevent problems, you want to become aware of everyday habits that create muscular imbalance, and for that, let's turn to a list compiled by fitness professional Beverly Hosford, working for the American Council on Exercise:

Sleeping on the same side every night. If you always sleep on one side, or on your stomach with your head always turned the same way, switch sides. At first, it will feel odd. Explore that sensation. Remind yourself that you're on a path to a more balanced body. Then, let go into dreamland.

Always leading with your dominant side when climbing. It's all about growing awareness. What foot leads going up stairs, and what foot leads going down? Pay attention, and do what we're always doing in yoga to stay in muscular balance—switch to the opposite side.

Crossing your legs with the same leg on top. If you cross your knees or ankles when you sit, notice which leg sits on top. Do the old switcheroo.

Carrying bags on the same shoulder. Which shoulder do you normally use to carry stuff—groceries, kids, computer bags? Consciously shift your load to the other shoulder. What does *that* feel like? If you ever feel pain, stop. If you feel your shoulder is hunched and tense, release. Experiment with smaller loads, both sides.

Using the same hand to hold things. Which hand holds your phone, your fork, your toothbrush? Switch from time to time. This crossover trick is also good for your brain, breaking up old patterns, sparking new pathways. Will it feel odd? Will some toothpaste miss the mark? I'm into my third week of switching my tooth brushing to my left hand instead of my right, and it still feels weird every time. So what? My brain is loving it.

Always putting your weight on one leg while standing. News flash! You're not an ostrich. So where is your weight when you're standing or leaning? To distribute the weight evenly over both feet, stand tall, your legs hip-width apart, and close your eyes. Shift your weight left and right, front to back, and settle into balanced, relaxed weight distribution from your feet to your head.

Locking your knees. Keep your knees soft when standing. Locking means you're blocking the flow of energy. Unlocked knees are happy knees, juicy knees, and when they're connected energetically to your feet, ankles, hips, and shoulders, alignment happens effortlessly. Relaxed and balanced muscles allow more energy to flow throughout your body. Tune into that feeling. Gently hug your muscles to your bones, and let that little pumping action flood every cell with juice and joy.

Holding your phone or tablet at waist level. "Text neck" is the next big thing in preventable, debilitating injuries. We all do it to see the screen—head down, neck scrunched, shoulders slouched—and we all will suffer the consequences unless we practice profound stretching and radical rebalancing in between.

One-sided training in sports. For this one, just picture Rafael Nadal's forearm. Tennis, golf, and bowling are sports that obviously overdevelop one side of the body. Assess your sport for one-sidedness, and correct the imbalance with focused weight training and cross-training, too.

Too much driving. Sit so your spine is aligned, your sacrum even, your shoulders relaxed. Take stretching breaks. Make tiny adjustments—mentally and physically—so your body is driving in a balanced, alert way.

That's it. It's all about bringing your body into balance, working both sides, back to front, up one side and down the other.

It's up to you. It's your body, your responsibility. Yes, it will take time to train yourself to tune in to your spine, your hips, your ankles before a twinge becomes a Tylenol special, but it's worth it. Isn't it?

So, remember this: Body awareness leads to self-care, and self-care prevents injuries and sustains personal well-being.

Okay! Class dismissed, and as you walk away, please notice which leg is in the lead.

ENERGY EXPRESS-O! Keep the Faith

"If you think you are too small to make a difference, try sleeping with a mosquito."
—Dalai Lama

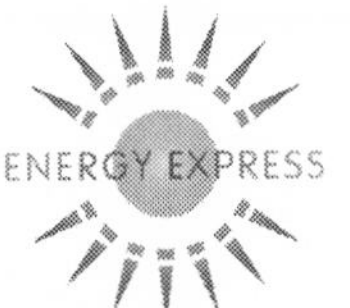

GOING DEEPER

The body is self-healing, but you can help it happen by developing your inner body awareness. Here are three magical words to help you: Concentration. Irrigation. Celebration.

Concentration is key. It means you pay attention, you focus your mind's eye and your breath on whatever area of the body you're hoping to reach.

Irrigation is transformative. It means your movements are spreading nourishing fluid and energizing blood throughout your body. This is a very good thing to do to your joints, muscles, tissues, and every cell in your body.

And celebration is what comes after you've done the first two things—concentration and irrigation—because it feels so good to move mindfully. And it helps prevent and recover from injuries, too.

So, now pick one activity you do every day—sitting, standing, driving, walking—and ask yourself:

As I do this particular thing, where is my body in space? Where do I feel tension? Where do I feel freedom? Is my spine aligned? Am I locking my knees? Am I standing with more weight on my right leg than my left?

Be curious. Pay attention. Don't judge. Your mind and your body are in this together. You just have to connect physically, mentally, energetically.

And you have to do this time and time again, day after day, patiently building a practice you can come back to all your life.

Awareness is first; taking action is second. Your victory dance comes later.

I couldn't get a massage during early COVID, so I dreamt about it instead. One time, I was on the table, and Nathan's magic fingers were buried deep in my lungs, and he said, "Look what I found, Marilynn," and he pulled out a 1967 Ford Mustang, my first car. Lots of people think getting a relaxing, rejuvenating massage is a selfish luxury. It's not. It's what self-care feels like. Sure, it costs money, but so do addictive pain relievers and unnecessary surgeries. Why do most insurance companies pay a hospital $50 for a box of tissues and refuse to reimburse you for a gifted body worker who releases tension, nourishes your muscles, and leaves you floating in a tub of butter? This pisses me off! But after a few minutes of deep pressure on the soles of my feet, all is well again.

Breathe In, Bliss Out.

I love a good massage. I even love a mediocre massage. I know there are people who can't stand being touched, and I respect that. But I also think they're nuts.

The older we get, the more we need wise and healing hands working us over, sensing our tight spots, stimulating blood flow, easing open the stuck places.

Sixty minutes is never enough. I'm an expert in healthy lifestyles. I believe in moderation, absolutely, but not when it comes to something as splendid for your body and mind as a massage. It's like crunchy peanut butter on a firm banana—the more, the better.

Where do you hold tension? It's always a good idea to let your body worker know your personal preferences. I'm an absolute glutton for glute work. A mauled bun is a happy bun. Out, damned knot! The more you can let go of tension in your buttocks and lumbar spine, the less likely you are to experience low back pain.

Massage equals prevention. In the best of all possible

worlds, just now coming, massage therapy would be part of our regular maintenance routines, like having our teeth cleaned or our hairs cut.

Skilled body workers do things for us that need to be done, especially as we age. They relieve aching muscles, soothe joint pain, help prevent sports injuries, and release energy blocks—physical and emotional—that keep us from living our healthiest, happiest life.

Many styles, many smiles. There is no one best massage technique. Massage is where the expression "different strokes for different folks" originated. Some of us like deep trigger-point work; others prefer lighter, longer strokes. And some like a sumo wrestler to dance on their spines.

No matter your choice—from hot stones to deep tissue, from Swedish to shiatsu—here are some suggestions that will make your next massage your best massage:

—**Go guilt-free.** Why lie there feeling guilty about the time or the money, when you could be congratulating yourself on your inner wisdom? Open up fully to the experience you are having. Stay in the moment while listening to whatever soothing music calms your busy brain and slows your breath.

—**Start with a scan.** Before your massage, scan your body for areas that feel tense or strained. Chronic soreness in your shoulder? Stiff neck? Tight quads? Tell your therapist, and then completely surrender to his or her touch. Engage your mind, ride the waves of your inhales and exhales, but let your therapist do the heavy lifting.

—**Settle into silence.** Avoid idle conversation. Talking about a new movie or an old lover is a distraction for both of you. But, of course, give feedback when necessary, especially about the amount of pressure you want. The more still you are, the more you can tune in to the experience.

—**Practice nasal breathing.** Take a few deep nasal breaths at the start to help you relax and get centered. If you begin to feel discomfort, don't clench or panic. Instead, direct your exhale to the area, and visualize the tension melting away. If it works, great. If not, don't be afraid to tell your body worker to ease up. The best ones will coach you to work with your breath during your session. Don't be shy about going with the flow, inhaling peace and joy, exhaling stress and credit card debt.

—**Unwind before, if possible.** A hot shower, bath, or sauna can start the unwinding process before the massage. And your therapist will appreciate a clean body to work with.

—**Enter lightly.** Don't come to the table with a full stomach. The less you have churning in your belly, the more comfortable you'll be. And remember to drink water afterward.

—**Be curious.** Before you leave the session, ask your therapist to tell you about particular areas of tension or imbalance. (It could be your neck, your shoulders, your hips.) That feedback can help you pinpoint areas that you need to work on when you're off the table.

(I know I'm repeating, but hear me: It's these tight, tense, stuck places that contribute to injuries and illness later on. Massage qualifies as superb self-care because it combines pleasure with prevention.)

Do-it-yourself massage works, too. If your budget is even tighter than your hamstrings, do what plenty of smart athletes do and learn to self-massage. Yoga, Qigong, and acupressure are splendid for that, and so is using a $25 foam roller, with good form and thoughtful guidance. A tennis ball can work, too, if you're willing to work it into the ball of your foot, the back of your shoulder, turning a nasty hot spot into a place of warmth and ease.

Once a month? Once a week? Whenever I'm on the table—not chewing over the past or worrying about the future—I'm thinking, why don't I do this more?

This really is what self-care feels like. And it's so much cheaper than a spinal fusion.

ENERGY EXPRESS-O! Use the Force

"When the body gets working appropriately,
the force of gravity can flow through.
Then, spontaneously, the body heals itself."
—Ida Rolf

ENERGY EXPRESS

GOING DEEPER

I'll bet you think I'm going to suggest you book yourself a massage this week.

Wrong.

Instead, reach for the oil of choice, and give someone you love your best version of a full-body massage.

If that stops you cold, hmmm…okay… make it a foot rub.

Set the scene. Clear the space and mark the moment in some special way, whatever that means to you. Light a candle. Ring a bell. Read a poem. Get in the mood, and pray your partner does, too.

Music definitely helps. So does dim light, no phones, and a deep dive into what your fingers are sensing as you massage the head, neck, shoulders, back, legs, arms, hands, and a twenty-five-point penalty if you forget the feet.

If I've just lost you because your loved one would kill you and move to the Outer Hebrides if you tried anything like this, then okay, book a massage for yourself. Book ten.

The human touch. We need it. There's nothing like it. Being without intimacy and touch has made the cost of COVID about a hundred times worse. Zooming and virtual reality will try to substitute, but don't be fooled. Humans need to feel connections to other humans if we want to stay healthy and strong, physically and mentally.

That's what we all want, right?

That's what every person on the planet deserves, right?

That's not political, is it?

Day after day, all during COVID, our most trusted public health officials talked about ways you could protect yourself from the virus. Wear a mask! Wash your hands! Stay at home! Social distance! Get the vaccine! I understand why all this advice was given. What I don't understand is this: Why weren't our honored medical authorities also telling us how to boost our immune system? Even now, why aren't they saying more about prevention? And treatment? When are simple and effective breathing practices going to be part of our recovery plan? There is solid science behind the fact that it's never too late to strengthen your immune system. I repeat: It's never too late to sleep more, stress less, exercise, eat real food, breathe properly, and cut out the overly processed foods that make us sick and weak and fat. This sound medical advice was ignored, forgotten, and, in some cases, openly mocked. Why is that? Our public health officials are well-intentioned, and when they neglect to talk about self-care, they are sabotaging the health of the whole country. I was shocked, confused, and deeply, wildly disappointed. And by the way, self-sabotage isn't good either.

Resist the Dark Forces.

Is exercise good for you?

Duh.

Regular workouts give you strength, energy, a trimmer body, a healthier heart, a calmer mind, and a much lower risk of at least thirty-five (!) different devastating diseases, including high blood pressure, stroke, osteoporosis, nonalcoholic fatty liver disease, diverticulitis, Type 2 diabetes, colon and breast cancer, and, yes, even that star of prime-time TV ads: erectile dysfunction.

In spite of what we know, we don't do. According to the latest research, ninety-two percent of adolescents and ninety-five percent of adults in the U.S. do not meet the minimum guidelines for physical activity.

Oh, dear. When I think about the gap between what we know about the benefits of exercise versus how much we actually do, my heart sinks, and my brain seizes.

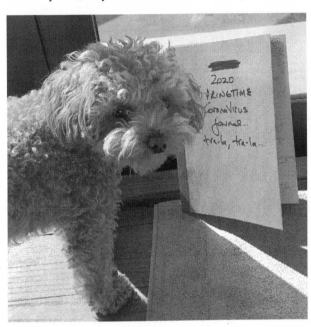

And then I remember the principles of self-sabotage and know I can be helpful. Once you understand that there's a right way and a wrong way to approach exercise, your days as a self-saboteur are over.

Do it grudgingly, on remote control, impatient for quick results, and you are setting yourself up to fail. Do it consciously, finding pleasure, forgiving lapses, and your chances of lifelong success are greatly improved.

Here are some typical ways we humans sabotage our own health and wellness, and what to do instead:

You aren't truly committed. Saying you want to get in shape is not enough. You've got to have a deep-down, nothing-will-stop-me commitment. Change will happen only when you are ready, and when you are—halleluiah!—not only will you be able to overcome every obstacle; you will actually enjoy the process.

You have failed before. Many people don't understand that change is not linear. It's often two steps forward, one step back. Exercise dropouts have failed before, and the fear of failing again often makes them quit. You can break this self-defeating cycle by taking fear of failure off the table. See failure as feedback. Know you can succeed, and you will succeed, if you are patient, persistent, and always practicing self-compassion.

You punish yourself instead of rewarding yourself. Negative self-talk will derail you. Listen to your inner voice. If it says you're lazy, stupid, ate too much, and can't get to the gym today, pay no attention. The mind attaches to the negative. It's your job to shift your thought to the positive. (Your body will follow because it can't not.) Start a new inner dialogue based on kindness and compassion for the healthier, happier person you want to be. Create positive affirmations, not unlike my favorite, "All is well," and repeat them often.

You compare yourself to others. Your best pal runs half-marathons, and you struggle with a 10K. Wendy can cycle forty miles, and you can barely finish twenty. So what? Jealousy and envy are counterproductive and will lead you astray.

Run your own race at your own pace, and you'll be setting your own records, reaching your own goals. When you see others who are stronger, more flexible, thinner, or more athletic, be happy for them. Find your serene smile, and return your focus to your own situation. Be grateful you have a situation.

You refuse to keep a journal. Journals may strike you as a homework assignment you refuse to do, but the truth is keeping a daily journal is a great tool for creating awareness and staying on track.

Please try it. Whatever you write is right: what you did, how long you did it, how you felt. What you write isn't as important as just doing it, every day.

Once you have the exercise habit in place, you can stop with the journaling, but if it does become a habit, journaling can be a powerful tool for transformations of all sorts.

(Keeping a self-care journal during COVID saved me from even more misery than I experienced, but I know you can't tell someone else what to do. Well, you can, but then you have to let go of the results. Do what you want, dear reader. But if you are ready to make a lifestyle change happen—more exercise, smarter eating, daily calming practices—get that journal going from Day One.)

You expect quick results. Impatience is a big problem for people just starting to exercise regularly. You expect immediate results, and when you don't see them, you find a reason to quit. Outsmart yourself. Take it day by day. Find joy in just showing up. In time, all the benefits of regular exercise will come your way. It takes the time it takes.

You see yourself as the victim. Many exercise dropouts blame their failure on someone or something else: I can't take time away from my kids; my job is too demanding; I travel too much.

These are excuses created to test your true intention. When you take responsibility for your own health and wellness, you give up being a victim and start living the more active, balanced, joyful life you've always wanted.

The beauty of self-sabotage is that whatever you do, you can undo. No guilt, no shame, just a willingness to begin again from where you are—this time with a new, improved attitude and greater understanding about what it takes to succeed.

ENERGY EXPRESS-O! Be a Selfie

"Be yourself; everyone else is already taken."
—Oscar Wilde

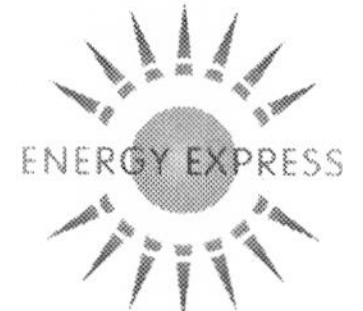

GOING DEEPER

Affirmations can sound corny.

"I love and approve of myself."

"I breathe in calmness and breathe out fear."

"I surround myself with people who treat me well."

And yet, they're popular and powerful. You can find hundreds of ready-made affirmations by searching online. Or you can make up your own.

Here's one that Venee McGee made up. She's the founder of Ebb & Flow Collective, a group of teachers and healers who help people on the soul path to life-changing self-care.

"I am open and receptive to the abundance of the Universe. I trust in you, I trust in me, for we are one. And I am grateful."

Do affirmations change lives? Absolutely. It did for Venee, from victim to warrior, she says, and it can for you.

You won't know until you experiment with a few phrases that feel good to you.

"All is well" always calms me and makes me smile. I didn't invent it, but it suits me, so I adopted it as my own early on.

"I can't do this" is a great example of what not to say.

"I'm too tired to go for a walk" is also a no-no. Change your thoughts; change your life.

Spinal twists sound like something to avoid. Who wants to twist a knee? An ankle? But spinal twists are different. Done gently, with awareness, they juice up your spine so it stays nourished, supple, spacious, and pain-free. Yoga poses were created to bring energy and freedom to your spine. It's not the only path to a more fluid spine, but it's been a good one for millions of practitioners, including me. Your path will be your path. I will say, after reporting on medical trends and tragedies for more than forty-five years, if our U.S. medical doctors understood what skillful yogis teach about the value of mindful movement and conscious breathing, I'm positive we'd all be healthier, happier, and much more involved with our own healing. We might also have more tattoos.

Twist and Soak.

I try not to talk about yoga with my friend Wendy because she's started and stopped Hatha yoga so many times. It's not for me, she says, and I accept that. Absolutely. But this time, I couldn't resist. I was doing research.

"What do you think's the purpose of all those twisting poses?" I asked.

"I have no idea," she said. "Stretching my laterals?"

So many smart people just think of yoga as what the poses look like on the outside, focusing on the external form: Triangle, Half-Moon, Down Dog.

Just as important—more important, really—is what is going on *inside* your body as you relax into each pose, creating space with your breath, directing energy in ways that restore muscle strength, fluidity, and balance.

Why twist? When you do a twist, as part of a pre-game warmup or a post-workout cooldown, you are giving many vital body parts a good squeezing. Followed by a good soaking. This revitalizes your organs, glands, muscles, and joints.

Your kidneys, your adrenals, your liver…different postures work different areas, but the one thing all twists have in common is that they flush out stagnant blood and bring in fresh, healing blood.

Twists bring oxygen and vital fluids to your spine, your hips, and your pelvis. Without that extra effort, as the body ages, many body parts shrivel and get stiff and painful from dryness and disuse.

Now, hear this: A collapsing spine and a stiff torso can be prevented. A few twists a day—breathe and squeeze!—really can help keep the doctor away. The back surgeon, too.

Learn how. So, now you know why you *should* do twists. Next, you need to learn *how*. A sensitive, experienced yoga teacher is one good place to begin.

I've learned from some great ones—deep bows to Tias Little, Sienna Smith, Jo Lewzey, Sarah Steen, Djuna Devereaux, Suddha Wexler—but many teachers I've met along the way weren't nearly as wise or skilled with their cues and instruction.

And please don't think that speeding up your yoga to keep up with your teacher is helping you develop a felt sense of what's going on inside your body. For that, you need to slow down and work with a teacher who understands the value of cultivating body awareness.

When that awareness is part of your practice, healing can happen. Without it, you can lurch your way into sprains, tears, and a very twisted understanding of why yoga is famous for harmonizing and strengthening mind and body.

Self-care. You don't want to over-twist, so it's your job to tune in to your body and respect your limits. Every twist isn't safe for everyone. It's one thing to go to your edge; it's another to push through pain. Never do that! And don't let an overly aggressive yoga teacher do it to you.

Now that you're revved up about twisting, why not give it a try?

Susan Winter Ward has written a useful book called *Yoga for the Young at Heart: Accessible Yoga for Every Body*. She describes a twist that "lubricates and nourishes the spinal column, increases elasticity of the muscles and ligaments of the spine, balances the nervous system; prevents backache, massages internal organs, toning liver, kidneys and spleen. Aids digestion and elimination."

Amazing! You can't say that about bowling.

What to do. "Sit on the floor, legs out in front of you. Bend your left knee and place your left foot on the floor to the outside of your right thigh. If you feel pain, don't continue. If you continue, ease into the twist slowly, mindfully, feeling your way."

Ward continues: "Inhale deeply as you extend your right arm out to the side, shoulder height.

"Exhaling, bring it around your left knee, holding your knee with the inside of your elbow. Draw the right side of your rib cage toward your inner left thigh.

"Inhale as you raise your left arm up and overhead. Keep your back flat and your heart lifted.

"Exhaling, lower your left hand to the floor behind you, as close to your tailbone as you can. Press the palm of your hand into the floor, lengthening your spine."

More instruction:

"Be sure that both sitting bones stay squarely on the floor.

"Inhale as you lift through the crown of your head and exhale as you rotate your chin to gaze over your left shoulder.

"Press against the floor to lengthen your spine with each inhalation and gently twist a bit more—if possible—with each exhalation, using your front arm and leg as a point of leverage.

"Take three to five long, slow inhalations and exhalations.

"Come out of the pose gently, inhaling as you raise your left arm overhead and exhaling as you bring your body around to face forward again.

"Take a few breaths, and repeat on the other side."

Twists are part of yoga because squeezing and soaking is so good for your body. Once you understand that, you'll find a zillion variations to try—on the floor, in a chair, standing at your desk.

Wherever and whenever you twist, do it with a sense of play and exploration. And do it breathing in and out of your nose, not your mouth.

Some days, you'll feel tight and tense. Other days, you'll feel free and fluid. Accept wherever you are that day; let go of expectations; and be happy you've taken the time to nourish the one and only body you'll ever have.

ENERGY EXPRESS-O! Soak Up the Gratitude

"When you arise in the morning, think of what a privilege it is to be alive—to breathe, to think, to enjoy, to love."
—Marcus Aurelius

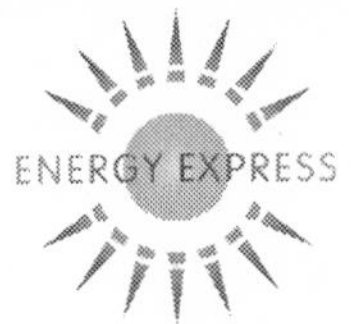

GOING DEEPER

Become a champion visualizer and your personal well-being will benefit in many magical ways. So will your tennis game, your running time, your breast stroke, and on and on to gardening, biking, skiing…

So, picture your spine.

I mean *really* picture it.

In your mind's eye, see your twenty-four stacked vertebrae (small bones of the spine); the soft, gel-like cushions called discs that tuck between each vertebrae; the ligaments that connect the bones to the bones; the tendons that connect the muscles to the bones.

Don't strain to memorize anything or make it perfect. Just see it the best you can; pat yourself on your latissimus dorsi; and refine your visualizing abilities over time, using whatever anatomy guides you prefer.

Each vertebra has a hole in the center so when they all stack up, they form a hollow tunnel that protects the entire spinal cord and its nerve roots.

Imagine your thirty-one pairs of nerve roots inside the spinal canal and all the nerve tissue that carries crucial and complex messages from your brain to everywhere else in your body.

And don't stop there. Picture the upper part, the cervical spine, with its seven vertebrae; and the central portion of the spine, the thoracic spine, with its twelve vertebrae; and the lower or lumbar portion, made up of five or six vertebrae. And just below that is your sacrum, yearning to be free.

Sensing a little complexity here? No wonder pain along the spine is so common, so difficult to treat with drugs that disguise the symptoms and do nothing to re-organize and re-balance the body.

Let's return our third-eye focus to the spine, and the four

basic curves—that's right, four!—and the fact that we depend on our spines to support our body, protect our central nerves, and move us about the planet in remarkable ways.

Once your visualization of your spine and how it moves is clear, and you're able to touch into it with your breath, your ability to boost your well-being will improve mightily.

And you'll never be bored when you're doing a twist or a stretch of any sort, anywhere, not just in a yoga class. You'll be focused on positioning yourself to bring energizing fluid to every organ, bone, and body part.

Picture that. A flexible spine, an open heart, a strong healthy back for the rest of your life. Wow.

I have a highly developed aversion to too much technology. I don't judge others who indulge, and I couldn't live the interesting and blessed life I do without the internet. But here's the truth: I spend as little time on my devices as possible. I have never tweeted or used an emoji. I create some amount of content for Instagram and Facebook because I know I should, but I depend on a skilled creative team at BadDog Design to do the actual posting. My neighbor's golden doodle has more followers than I do. I know I shouldn't be shunning social media, especially with a book to promote. I'm being authentic, I tell myself. Moderation in all things. Is it a pathology or past lives? Do I need an intervention?

Tweet Mindfully.

Whenever I see someone texting while driving—Stop that! Pull over, you idiot!—I start to worry about the cumulative impact of social networking on our brains, our bodies, our fenders, and our nondigital pursuit of a healthy lifestyle.

Tweeting forty times a day. Texting fifty times a day. Nonstop checking of emails in between. It's a huge time suck, that's for sure. And "not enough time" is the No. 1 excuse people use for eating poorly and not exercising.

But wait! Going online is not the enemy. The internet is a window to the biggest, most fascinating world we've ever known. Tweeting has its upside and downside: It discourages empathy and dumbs down deep thinking, but it carries tremendous influence and can work to connect and lift the spirits of people fighting for freedom and justice. Facebook fosters instant, global connections at the same time it redefines and degrades what it is to be—truly, intimately—a friend.

And let's please not veer off into the terrifying subject of social media and censorship. It's so complicated. But I'm too young to go back to the quill pen. I have to face up to my confusion and struggle to find the middle way between too much social media and not enough. We all do. And that's why I found Lori Deschene's tweeting advice in *Tricycle* magazine so helpful.

(Tweeting tips in a major spiritual magazine? Absolutely. Remember, it was the Buddha who said, "If you propose to speak, always ask yourself, is it true, is it necessary, is it kind.")

Deschene believes in using social media mindfully, as opposed to endlessly. Are you obsessively addicted to email? Do you feel too tied to technology? Are you squeezed for time to live the life you want? Here are some of Deschene's guidelines to help you calm your brain, save your thumbs, and get back in balance:

Practice letting go. It may feel unkind to ignore some tweets or updates, but to be kind to ourselves, we need downtime—time away from technology. Give yourself permission to let yesterday's stream go by, to come to the dinner table without being tethered to your phone.

Be your authentic self. Text/tweet/email about the things that really matter to you. If you need advice or support, ask for it. Ego-driven tweets focus on an agenda; authenticity communicates from the heart.

Offer random tweets of kindness. Every now and then, Deschene asks on Twitter, "Is there anything I can do to help or support you today?" It's her way of connecting personally to followers, her way of giving to others without any expectations in return.

Experience now; share later. Next time you're inclined to snap a picture with your phone, upload it to Instagram, or email it to a friend, pause and reflect: This is keeping me from being in the moment. The less digital narration, the more present you can be. Can you do both? Maybe, but the present moment will suffer.

Be active, not reactive. Instead of having your day constantly interrupted by activity alerts on your social media accounts, decide to choose when and if you want to join the conversation. "Don't expect me to respond to this (email, text, tweet) after 7 p.m. at night" is how one friend of mine handles it.

Enjoy social media. Social media is here to stay. Our job is to use it in a way that helps us feel present and purposeful, not obsessed and addicted. Follow your instincts. If you're a mindful person when you're disconnected from technology, you have all the tools you need to be mindful when you go online.

If these tips sound good to you but you're not sure how to start, follow the advice of Tim Ferriss, the celebrated author of *The 4-Hour Workweek*, a smash hit of a book that has some very good ideas about how to make life less stressful.

To cope with the constant crush of email, Ferriss suggests you set up an automatic reply that tells senders you only check your inbox twice a day, at noon and at 4 p.m. Or copy this:

"Thank you for your email. Sadly, it will be deleted. To regain sanity, I am taking a break from email until March. If it is still relevant, please email me again in the month of March."

WHAT! What will people think?

Fear not. If they relax their overused thumbs and *do* think about it, they'll think you're getting your life back under control.

ENERGY EXPRESS-O! You Talking to Me?

"I am not anti-technology, I am pro-conversation."
—Sherry Turkle

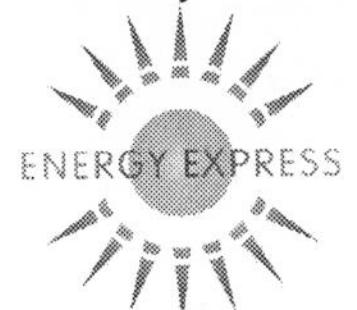

GOING DEEPER

Do you dare notice the amount of time you spend online?

Oh, go ahead. Be brave. Just for fun.

Keep track of how many texts you send in a day, how many times you check your email, how many games you play, videos you watch, social media stuff you post.

It's a cruel thing to ask, I know.

But do it. Just for a day. If possible.

And if it isn't possible, sit back and notice that.

There is a war against breast cancer—and at the same time, there is a battle against the war on breast cancer. All that "pink washing" has some people seeing red. Too many nonprofits and businesses are fueling their own growth while the growths that turn into breast cancers continue to affect astonishing numbers of women, and men, too. And now medical authorities tell us that mammograms aren't really useful when it comes to preventing breast cancer and are causing more harm than good. Oops. This is a hot topic for me and every woman I know, which is why it's time to...

Warm Up to Thermograms.

Breast cancer doesn't just run in my family; it gallops. My grandmother, my mother, my sister, my niece, and way too many more women I know and love have all been diagnosed. So, when I tell you I keep abreast of this subject, you'll know I'm not just punning you.

And here's what I've discovered about the war on breast cancer that is crucial and has nothing to do with the color pink: Women should take command of their bodies and include thermograms as part of their breast health regimen.

Don't wait for your gynecologist or primary doctor to suggest it. Chances are they know nothing about this continually improving imaging technology. It's had lousy PR ever since it was approved by the FDA in 1982. Maybe that's because it's simply not part of the multibillion-dollar cancer industry. Maybe people would pay more attention if thermography had a color of its own. What about gold?

Breast thermography—using a state-of-the-art digital infrared camera—is safe, effective, involves no radiation or squishing of the breast, and is evolving as a super-important risk-assessment tool for the early detection of breast cancer.

And early detection is everything. "When treated in its

earliest stages, most breast cancer has a cure rate of ninety-five percent," says Dr. Kathryn Ater, a Doctor of Oriental Medicine, who gave me my first, second, and third thermograms over the last several years.

Her mission is simply stated on her Two Birds Thermography website, thermographynewmexico.com: to help women take care of themselves.

"You are the one who decides when and how you're going to monitor your breast health," says Dr. Kate, who's been analyzing thermograms for more than ten years. "Thermography is a tool. It's a piece of the puzzle that we can offer to help find abnormalities in the breast tissue before abnormal growth begins."

Mammograms—and I'm not going to get into all the pros and cons that have women so confused—are simply not useful for early detection.

"A cancer has been growing eight to ten years before it's big enough or dense enough to be detected by mammography," explains Sandra Fields, a Certified Clinical Thermographer with a master's in nursing and thirty-five years of experience in women's health care. She's part of an expanding network of doctors, nurses, patients, and health experts who are spreading the good word about thermograms.

"Women need to know that breast thermography is a promising and safe technology that is a welcome addition to helping women create breast health," says another wise advocate, the bestselling author Dr. Christiane Northrup.

The science is simple and makes sense to anyone with a breast or a brain: By the time a tumor is the size of a pinhead (after about two years of growing), it requires its own blood supply. The process of developing that blood supply is called angiogenesis. Thermography is the best technology for detecting angiogenesis because it detects abnormal activity in the breast—increased heat, blood flow, or changing vascular patterns. All of these are early indicators that something suspicious is happening in the breast tissue and needs follow-up.

It's an easy, painless procedure that takes about thirty minutes. The patient stands naked from the waist up, turning in different directions while the technician clicks away, using an infrared thermal camera.

I felt relieved when Dr. Kate went over my most recent thermogram with me. We both looked at the beautiful result, worthy of framing, a swirling psychedelic Peter Max-like pattern of red, blue, green, and yellow.

"Looks good," are the words I remember. She compared the new one with the one from last year. No new vascular supply, no suspicious heat patterns, no new asymmetries.

"Nothing's really changed," she said, and we both knew that was very good news.

I'm not waiting for my insurance company to do the right thing. I pay the $199 out of pocket, and $50 more for Dr. Kate's careful review of the results.

I'm not saying that a thermogram can or should replace a mammogram. You must decide for yourself. But it is an accurate and reliable first line of defense and prevention, an excellent tool for early detection of a spreading blood supply, and it's not getting the good publicity it merits.

"Why is that?" I ask myself. I know the answer, and it's frustrating and doesn't help spread the word about thermograms.

What will?

ENERGY EXPRESS-O! Picture This!

"With thermography as your regular screening tool, it's likely that you would have the opportunity to make adjustments to your diet, beliefs, and lifestyle to transform your cells before they become cancerous. Talk about true prevention."
—Christiane Northrup, M.D.

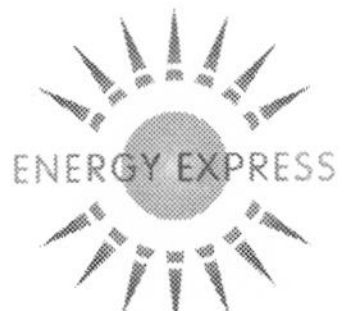

GOING DEEPER

Breast cancer is a subject very near and dear to my heart. Yours, too, probably. Everyone knows someone.

I've made my case. My readers will decide for themselves whether or not to pursue thermography.

But here's another way to go deeper into alleviating the breast cancer epidemic. You can support prevention by helping girls develop into healthy, strong, confident women, with a lower risk of breast cancer and other cancers, too.

You can engage in what I call fitness philanthropy and support an amazing nonprofit called Girls in the Game.

GIG changes lives one girl at a time. It started in my hometown of Chicago in 1995 with the mission of helping girls in underserved communities find their voice and develop into leaders. The girls do that by playing sports and learning about wellness, yoga, breathing, and other self-care strategies that help them handle the stress and trauma that comes with the neighborhood.

GIG's success is well documented, badly needed, and models excellence when it comes to inspiring hope and health at a community level.

"Girls in the Game understands that not all playing fields are equal," you can read on their website, "hence our vision is for a world where all girls are empowered to be gamechangers."

There's plenty of data to show that girls who grow up eating smart, exercising regularly, and learning healthy ways to handle anger and depression can lower their risk for developing breast cancer later in life, especially if they get motivated to avoid obesity.

In GIG's twenty-five-plus years, we've had great success working with girls from ages seven to eighteen, not just during school but also at our remarkable life-affirming summer camp.

I say "our" because I was the founding chair of GIG, and I'm still a shameless board member.

So, go deeply into GirlsintheGame.org, and please support us with time, money, love. Pay special attention to a program I helped start with Venee McGee, called the Self Care Project: https://support.girlsinthegame.org/campaign/teens-self-care-project/c342954.

It has its own fundraising page on the GIG website, and as you know from this book, one of the best ways to feel good yourself is to do good for others.

Told you I was shameless.

One of the saddest developments of the last forty-five years is the ginormous rise in childhood obesity. And yes, the stress and boredom and lunacy of COVID made an unhealthy situation worse. Adults got fatter; kids got fatter; and we lost the opportunity to tell humans of all ages how they can help strengthen their immune systems with smart eating, more sleep, regular exercise. Why wasn't that part of the public health messaging? Instead, we continue to sell our children to the junk food vendors and sugary drink manufacturers, and—oh, boy and oh, girl—are they paying the price. In 2019, researchers reported that in the previous thirty years, the prevalence of childhood obesity had more than doubled, and it tripled in adolescents. Now, about one in three American kids and teens is overweight or obese. All that excess weight puts innocent kids at much greater risk of heart disease, diabetes, cancer, low self-esteem, depression, and early death. It's a national disgrace, and even the best and brightest intentions of former first lady Michelle Obama weren't enough to make Big Food and Big Soda reform their naughty ways. So, here's a bit of good news to focus on: Some kids are fighting back.

Let Them Eat Rice Cakes.

It can happen in the best of homes. You think you've done everything right as a parent—good schools, restricted screen time, all-cotton underwear—and then, one day at dinner, your world explodes.

Your kid goes veggie. She stops eating meat. "I've decided on a plant-based diet," Emma announces out of the blue, turning up her nose, knife, and fork at the beautiful burger on her plate. "How can you eat somebody's mother?"

Some version of this drama plays out every day in homes across America as more young people become aware of the face on the plate and how it relates to the planet they live on. If you want to help reduce climate change, you have to eat like it matters, because it really does.

Which is why kids eating green is trending up, and meatloaf-loving parents need help, strategies, patience, sometimes pharmaceuticals.

Step one? Don't panic. There are experts to advise you, and one of them is Lisa Barley, writing in *Vegetarian Times*, a great resource for one hundred things to do with chickpeas.

"Your child's new diet doesn't have to make your life more difficult," she explains in language meant to calm you. There are ways to be supportive, less stressed. Here are some of them, along with my own embellishments:

Don't worry. Your kids' health won't suffer if they're following a well-planned veggie diet, say the authorities, including the American Academy of Pediatrics. They can get all the vitamins and minerals they need to be healthy and strong, but it requires some study and effort. Open up to wiser ways of eating and you will benefit, too.

Listen up. Ask your kids to share the reasons they're giving up meat, Lisa suggests. Keep an open mind. If they've gone on YouTube and seen the horrible things that happen to cows and chickens in the name of factory farming, take a look yourself. Sit down over a plate of edamame, and talk it over. More important than talking is *listening* to your child. Listening without judging.

"Think of it as an opportunity to get to know their values and worldview," Lisa Barley writes.

Assign homework. Lisa wants you to get your kids involved in whatever eating changes they want to make. Have your newbie vegetarian "make a list of nutritious snacks and meals and draft a shopping list," she says in a state of mind some parents will regard as delusional.

Another strategy: Go over the vegetarian food pyramid together so all involved can see what a well-balanced diet looks like. In case your vegetarian food pyramid has gone missing, you can always find it again at http://www.vegetariannutrition.org/6icvn/food-pyramid.pdf.

Be a student. When a child goes veggie, it's smart to have a couple of reliable resources you can turn to with your questions and concerns. But beware! There is a lot of confusing, conflicting, and corporately designed nutrition information online. Keep your focus on plant food, not food made in a plant. Lisa recommends parents check in with two nonprofits I've trusted and admired for years: Oldways Vegetarian Network and Physicians Committee for Responsible Medicine.

Set ground rules. Rule No. 1: "Make it clear that junk food vegetarianism won't fly," Lisa says. Eating real food should be the focus, not bags of chips and cookies that are marked vegan and packed with sugar. If you need help with meal planning and prep, ask your child to pitch in. (Why do I hear you laughing?)

And keep the drama over food choices to a minimum. Declare the dining table a no-war zone. Nothing puts a bigger chill in the air than a heated discussion about tortured and stressed industrial chickens...while half the family is chewing on them.

Cook and eat together. I've saved the best for last. It's also the most idealistic, but so what? Help create a world where everyone respects everyone else's food choices. Start in your own kitchen. Focus on foods you can all eat together, like make-your-own tacos with different fillings. Or pasta with one meat sauce, one veggie sauce. DIY pizza is good, too.

The crucial thing is your attitude. A kid choosing to go meatless isn't the end of the world. It's an introduction to a world you might want to join yourself someday.

As one mother told Lisa, "There are many bad choices that a child can make in this world, and being a vegetarian is definitely not one of them."

ENERGY EXPRESS-O! LOL

"Vegetarian—that's an old Indian word meaning lousy hunter."
—Andy Rooney

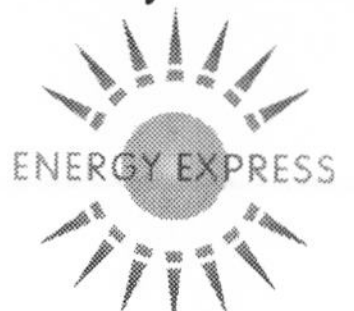

GOING DEEPER

Getting your young ones to make healthy food choices is right up there with climbing Mount Everest, in a bikini and high heels.

It's challenging. But it's not out-of-the-realm impossible. One strategy is to cozy up to your kid and read aloud from Michael Pollan's classic *Food Rules*, a small book that can have a huge impact on your entire family's eating habits and poundage. You can also bring it to the table one night and let everyone read a rule:

—"If it came from a plant, eat it; if it was made in a plant, don't."

—"It's not food if it arrived through the window of your car."

—"The whiter the bread, the sooner you'll be dead."

—"Eat animals that have themselves eaten well."

And what third-grader won't love this one?

—"Avoid food products containing ingredients that a third-grader can't pronounce."

Pollan's book works well for kids because he's written it in a simple and straightforward style, stripping away all the hard science, the biochemistry, the thermodynamically complex descriptions of insulin and fat metabolism.

Instead, he artfully delivers sixty-four rules that are fun to read and easy to digest. Maybe you can write the rules down on pieces of paper, put them into a jar, and draw one or two out at every meal.

Here are a few more samples, just to whet your appetite for the real thing:

"Eat (real) food." Every year, about 17,000 new products show up on grocery shelves, and most of them are so anti-health they shouldn't even be called food. Pollan calls them "edible food-like substances" and "industrial novelties." Avoid them, and watch how much better you feel.

"Avoid food products containing ingredients that no ordinary human would keep in the pantry." When was the last time you ran to the store for another box of ammonium sulfate? Or ethoxylated diglycerides? These additives are there to prolong shelf life, not your life. Stay away.

"Avoid foods that are pretending to be something they are not." Imitation butter, imitation (nonfat) cream cheese, soy-based mock meats…

Just say no.

And this final one:

"Don't eat breakfast cereals that change the color of your milk." Why? Because those are the cereals that are highly processed and full of refined carbohydrates and chemical additives.

What ten-year-old can resist seeing what happens with his next bowl of Coco Pops?

The slow-moving horror show we call COVID had many hidden blessings, and one of them involved the truth of impermanence. In or out of a pandemic, people die. Loved ones are heartbroken. This question lives on: How do you comfort the grieving? It's something to think about, learn about, offer up to friends who are suffering. One thing I know to be true in my forty-five years tracking healthy lifestyle habits is that the more you learn about death, the greater your joy in life. You feel liberated, unafraid to engage with the inevitable. You actually want to. Loving life isn't a state of denial, and death isn't the enemy; it's the star you navigate by to lead the life you'll leave.

Bring Life to Death.

Dealing with death—your own, a loved one's, the death of a child—is a required course at the University of Well-Being, Ballet, and Refrigeration.

No one gets out of here alive. This we know. What we don't know is everything else. Death is the biggest mystery of all, leaving many of us clueless when it comes to comforting someone who's lost a loved one.

What do you say? What *don't* you say? Do you mention the dead person by name? Do you try to offer good advice, to be helpful and loving?

"Do *not* give advice," advises Edie Hartshorne, a master of social work, longtime therapist, former Fulbright Scholar, and award-winning author of *Light in Blue Shadows*, a wise and inspiring book about death, compassion, and transforming grief.

After her twenty-year-old son, Jonathan, died unexpectedly, Edie went on a dark and deep journey into her own pain and unraveling. When she came out the other side and wrote her book—"a journey of loss and grief that leads to a place of wonder," says Isabel Allende on the jacket cover—Edie had a new awareness of many things, including what it means to comfort and be comforted.

"Many times when we feel uncomfortable with another person's loss, we offer advice, hoping to make everything better."

Resist, says Edie. The person grieving doesn't need advice. She needs to be heard, to have her loss acknowledged. She needs her friends, her family, to be fully present, listening to whatever she has to say.

Here are some more empowering Edie-isms to help you through the inevitable:

Don't say you know just how the grieving person feels. You don't! So don't equate or compare your grief to the other person's. When you say, "I know just how it is. I lost my mom a year ago," it can trivialize the other person's pain.

"This can be particularly true when a parent has lost a child," Edie writes. "It's better to make no comparisons."

Don't remain silent. Very often, because we fear saying the wrong thing, we say nothing at all about the truth of what's going on. That's a mistake, Edie counsels. It's isolating for the person who's grieving to be surrounded by silent friends.

"It's so important to validate the other person's reality," she writes. Share your truth plainly. "I just heard your terrible news. I am so sorry and sad. I just want you to know I am holding you in my heart." Say it your way, with your true voice, but don't hide in silence.

Don't try to fix your friend or family member. This goes along with "not giving advice," but you can't hear it often enough: "There is nothing to fix," Edie writes. It's natural for someone to feel grief when a loved one dies, and it's very painful.

Your work is to "stay present to the other person's pain." Just be there. It's not your job to solve anything.

Don't ask, "Is there anything I can do?" Just do it. Take the initiative. When people grieve, Edie says, they're often too overwhelmed to sort out what needs to be done or too shy to ask for help.

Notice what needs to be done, and take action: Bring over dinner; drop off flowers; walk the dog. This requires a sensitive touch, but if you wait to be asked, you may miss the opportunity to truly help.

Rather than focusing on the don'ts, embrace what you can do for your loved ones in times of grief. These do's are closer to Edie Hartshorne's true nature. She's a poet, a musician, and a very positive person:

Be present to exactly where your grieving friend is in the moment. If six months have passed and he suddenly bursts into tears, "take a deep breath to bring yourself fully into the moment," says Edie. "Listening fully and with a big heart is the most powerful medicine."

Make phone calls to your friend or family members during that first year. Grieving people are achingly aware of the birthdays and anniversaries involving the person who died. Say something! It feels very lonely when those dates go by unacknowledged.

ENERGY EXPRESS-O! Everything Changes

"Life and death are of extreme importance. Time swiftly passes by and opportunity is lost. Each of us should strive to awaken. Awaken! Take heed, do not squander your life."
—Eihei Dogen

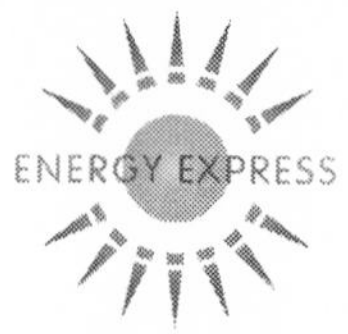

GOING DEEPER

The global pandemic suddenly brought so much death into our lives—in person, on our feed, a 24/7 parade of horribles—it was easy to forget that death is part of life.

All we could think about, day after dizzying day, was staying safe, staying home, wearing a mask, social distancing, and protecting our loved ones, because we wanted to stay alive and we didn't want them to die either.

And yet they did…way too many of them…so it's no wonder we're in the midst of a monumental, let us say existential, mental health crisis. Not only in America, but around the world.

To Go Deeper, go small. Do what Edie suggests: Simply call one friend or family member who's lost a loved one this past year.

It may be difficult for you, but don't let fear stand in the way. As I once heard Patti Smith say, "If you fear going to the next level, you'll never get to the next layer."

Make the call with the intention of listening, not talking.

Listen without interrupting.

Allow for silent moments, without feeling discomfort. Let the conversation unfold.

You're not calling to fix anything.

When you hang up, you'll feel very good that you made the call.

And so will your friend.

And that's what compassion looks like.

Autumn

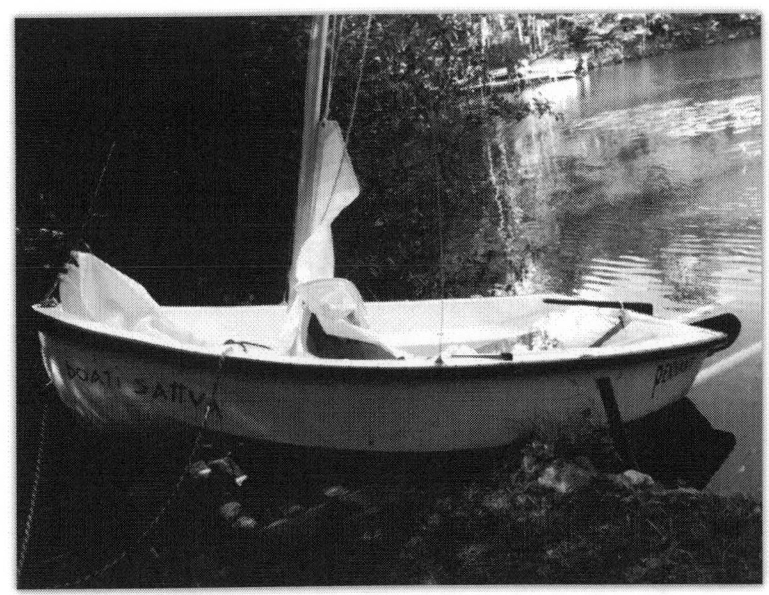

North Woods, Wisconsin

"Delicious Autumn!
My very soul is wedded to it, and if I were a bird
I would fly about the earth seeking
successive autumns."
—George Eliot

"Autumn calls us to a still and silent place and
beckons us to sit back and observe a little deeper."
—Natalie Goldberg

"There is something so special in the early leaves
drifting from the trees—as if we are all allowed a
chance to peel, to refresh, to start again."
—Ruth Ahmed

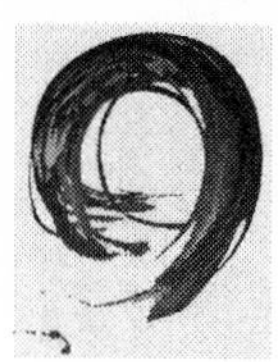

How do you maintain a healthy weight? It's so personal, so painful for so many. Not my mother. She was zaftig and beautiful, and she never tortured herself with diets. "Never go on a diet," she told me while I was still young enough to have her chocolate cake and milk for breakfast every day. "You'll only gain it all back and more." All the research on dieting has proven her right. I was a junior size 15-16 when I graduated from high school, and now I'm not. And that's because, eventually, I learned how truly wise my mother was. The chocolate cake for breakfast thing? No one's perfect.

Never Diet Again.

It's sad to see so many people in the country overweight and desperate, crippled and confused by the food they eat. It's the fake foods that make us fat, and the real foods that our bodies thrive on. Yet Big Food thrives on selling us cheap, manufactured fare, so obesity overtakes us, and we're left with crumbs.

What to do? Go see a nutritionist. This is what I find myself telling countless people—family, friends, total strangers on airplanes—in spite of all I know about the fruitlessness of giving advice. Add a nutritionist to your health team. A gifted body worker is good, too, but a savvy nutritionist is worth her weight in avocados.

Here's why it's so crucial: Your body chemistry—the building blocks of your health and well-being—is uniquely your own. Yes! Just like your fingerprints, only different, because your fingerprints stay the same, but your nutritional profile is something you can transform in weeks...if you really want to.

But you have to proceed with caution. We are constantly being seduced by what we see on TV, in magazines, online 24/7. Need strength? Swallow this powder! Energy? Take this multivitamin! A healthy microbiome? Swallow this glowing green drink!

Maybe you need supplements; maybe you don't. Just because your best friend takes calcium doesn't mean you need to. The only way to determine what nutrients to add or subtract is to discover what your body levels are right now.

High in cholesterol? Low in vitamin B-12? Getting enough vitamin D? Simple blood and urine tests will tell the tale. Eureka! Then what?

Chances are horrendously good that the doctors in your life don't know beans about nutrition. It's an uncomfortable truth, but we have to face it if we want to find our path to personal well-being. Food is medicine. If you don't feed your body the real food it needs—including the proper mix of nutrients, from antioxidants to zinc—it will, over time, underperform, get sick, and fall apart. It's that simple.

But figuring out how to get the nutrients we need to digest our food, support our hearts, nourish our brains, resist disease and inflammation, and promote good health and energy has become incredibly confusing.

If sugar is so lethal in excess—and it is—why is it packed into so many of our processed foods? Why is olive oil good and fake butter blends bad? Why is it so important to limit certain carbs and get your body to burn fat instead of glucose?

That's why a continuing relationship with a nutritionist is such a satisfying experience. The good ones can teach us which foods help us heal and which make us sick. They can help us help ourselves cut back on sugar and understand the importance of healthy fats. Together, you can fine-tune your body chemistry, using real food and drink instead of exotic fasts, expensive cleanses, and unnecessary supplements.

A skilled nutritionist also can tell you if you have any

imbalances—too acidic or too alkaline, too much iron or too little—and customize an eating plan that moves you toward better memory, a mightier metabolism, and fewer burps and belches.

So why isn't this kind of vital counseling commonly covered by our medical insurance? It's crazy! It's also an indication of how sick our drug-centered health care system is.

The Affordable Care Act looks a little more kindly on wellness and prevention, but overall, it's not really helping the ordinary citizen get on the path to personal well-being.

COVID showed us what an unhealthy country we've become, and now, as we pick up the pieces of a completely inadequate public health system, who knows how, when, or if we'll build back better.

Will kids learn to resist the junk and eat smarter? Can adults learn to prevent obesity, diabetes, depression with coaching strategies that we know work? Will the nation wake up to harm done to our hearts and guts by processed foods that sap our strength and clog our digestion?

I dream of it, but I don't see much evidence, not yet. That's why I keep reminding you that self-care is the best care, because only you can decide what you'll eat and what you'll let go of because it's no longer serving you and, even worse, it's making you sick.

You really *are* what you eat. Sit down with an experienced, enlightened nutritionist, and review your body chemistry, one on one, vitamin by mineral, protein by fat, so you can begin to understand the relationship between what you eat and how you feel, and what your body requires in terms of food to be strong, to be happy, to heal from illness and prevent disease.

Do not, I warn you, try this with your family doctor. I

know that's changing a tiny bit, but still, the vast majority of our docs still treat illness with drugs, not lifestyle change. It's hard to blame them, because that *is* what's taught in medical school. It's what drug companies prefer, too, but don't get me started on that or I'll never get back to the subject, which is this: If you want some clarity about what to eat to maintain a healthy weight and a fully functioning body, partner up with a nutritionist and learn what's right for you.

That said, I must now confess: Until a few years ago, I'd never been to one myself. I've interviewed them, gone to workshops, read their books, praised the role they play in wellness and weight control, but I'd never actually consulted with one—my body chemistry, her big brain—before.

And then I met professor Carmen Fusco, clinical nutritionist and research scientist, who has a remarkable understanding of the healing power of food. I nearly cried after my first two-hour session with her, and not just because I had to pay out-of-pocket. She's a genius!

And now I want everyone I know to find his or her own Carmen Fusco, assuming we can't clone her, which she wouldn't like at all.

ENERGY EXPRESS-O! This Is No Yolk

"Marilynn! Look at your white cell count. You're fighting a virus! I want you adding turmeric to your eggs!"
—Carmen Fusco

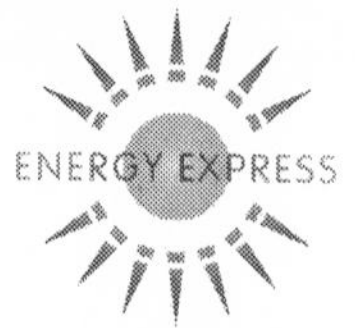

GOING DEEPER

When COVID-19 struck, overweight people had nowhere to hide. They were among the most vulnerable, the most dead, the least likely to get the self-care coaching they need.

Greg Hottinger and Michael Scholtz are two names that carry a lot of weight in the world of getting thinner… and staying thinner…if thinner is something you truly long to be.

They are both dieting experts, skillful coaches, and co-authors of what could be the last dieting book you'll ever need if, by some miracle, you follow their reasoning, stop undermining your own success, and pursue a kinder, gentler path to sustainable weight loss.

The path they've come to believe in isn't fixated on numbers on a scale or calories in a cookie. It's based on—hold on, now—self-acceptance, self-love, resiliency, and a deep understanding of how certain actions and beliefs are undermining your own success, whether or not you're conscious of it.

"*Coach Yourself Thin* is not an extreme or fad diet, nor is it an intimidating one-way-or-the-highway fitness plan," they write. "It is a guide that will help you identify the real-life obstacles that have been holding you back from losing weight."

What are those obstacles? In early 2021, I decided to take a deep dive into that question and signed up for an eight-week course with Greg and Michael to learn the latest about what works and what doesn't when it comes to losing weight, keeping it off, and finding joy and comfort in the process.

Here's a very thinned down version of three of their five stepping stones to lasting change:

1. Expect greatness. "The diet and exercise industry has been feeding you a lie," they write. "They want you to believe that real change is made only by people who have the 'right' plan or the 'best' exercise equipment—whatever it is they are currently trying to sell." Don't believe them. Instead, believe in yourself. Have faith in yourself and your ability to change. It takes work, discipline, patience, support, and a willingness to redefine success. "Expecting greatness," they write, "means you will bring to bear both a healthy dose of realism and an expansive imagination."

2. Regain your balance. In the aftermath of COVID (and in the before-math, too), we're suffering from too little sleep, too much processed food, too much stress, strained relationships, and "a Quick Fix Mindset that makes you question why you should have to give up your favorite chili dogs when you can just take an antacid an hour before you go to the ball game."

The first step to regaining your balance is to admit your life is out of balance. The second step is to take a healthy approach—not a Quick Fix mindset—to feeling better and losing weight. You regain your balance by protecting your "me time"—smart eating, enjoyable activities, seeing friends, feeling gratitude. "You may have to overcome the notion that 'me time' is inherently selfish," they write. "Taking care of your health is one of the most selfless things you can do."

3. Be unstoppable. Greg and Michael have heard every excuse in the book for not being able to lose weight. "My parents were fat… I have food allergies… My work schedule is impossible…"

Excuses are useless. They only get in the way of your success. "To overcome your excuses, real life challenges, and the undermining effects of negative emotions (disgust, anger, frustration), you'll need to become unstoppable," they write. That means you take control of your choices. You accept responsibility for their outcomes. You stop blaming others. You take back control.

And most powerful, you stop looking for perfection and accept yourself just the way you are. "Instead of waiting until you reach your goal weight to see the positives in your life, look for them now, be grateful for what you have, and watch how the door to change opens up."

Amen.

After forty-five-plus years on the fitness beat, and more than a year of living through the terrors of COVID-19, I've developed a healthy skepticism about medical care in the United States. It serves too few, costs too much, and discriminates against people of color and limited resources. Delivery can be cruel and downright sloppy. I'm not blaming our health care workers. They are angels. It's not their fault that our system is broken and needs nonpartisan repair. Preventable medical errors are the third leading cause of death in America—death from medical care itself! Our mainstream M.D.s are a mixed bag. Some can save your life. Others—think opioid epidemic—might kill you. Overmedicating is standard. To be wary is to be wise. I learned that and a whole lot more reading a fascinating book by the fearless and famous Dr. Jerome Groopman.

Team Up With Your Doctor.

Who likes going to the doctor? Exactly. No one…especially if you have something we all dread—symptoms!

A sudden chest pain, a nagging backache, a persistent headache. Though the symptoms will vary, your goal is always the same. You want your physician to figure out what's wrong. And you want to get well. Fast.

And that's why Dr. Jerome Groopman's award-winning classic, *How Doctors Think*, is so valuable. He teaches us to be a better patient. He recognizes that doctors are far from perfect. They make mistakes, and the majority of errors they make are not technical screwups, but rather errors in thinking.

Doctors are under great pressure to perform and perform quickly, Groopman explains. They jump to conclusions they're comfortable with. They ignore facts that don't fit. They have egos and emotions that can cloud their judgment and lead them astray. In short, they're just like us. Human.

So, how can you avoid those problems and hugely improve the quality of your medical care? Here are some highlights from *How Doctors Think*:

Be a partner. You can't be passive or shy or intimidated by your doctor. To lower your risk of a wrong diagnosis, Groopman says, you must be engaged and involved.

"Patients and their loved ones can be true partners with physicians when they know how their doctors think and why doctors sometimes fail to think."

Trust your instincts. If you sense your doctor is rushing through your exam or isn't listening to your story or just plain doesn't like you, pay attention.

"Research shows that patients do pick up on a doctor's negativity, but few understand how that affects their care, and they rarely change doctors." Groopman's advice? Change doctors!

Don't be pigeonholed. Doctors think in stereotypes: the hysterical housewife, the overworked executive, the kooky hypochondriac. If you think your doctor isn't paying enough attention to who you really are and what you're saying, call him or her on it.

Be informed. It's okay, even desirable, to learn everything you can about your case "and respectfully question each and every assumption about the diagnosis and treatment."

You do this not because you don't trust the doctor or hospital, Groopman writes, "but because God did not make people omniscient."

Ask questions. "What we say to a physician and how we say it sculpts his thinking. That includes not only our answers, but our questions."

You can positively influence your doctor's thinking by

asking smart questions: "What else could it be?" "Is there anything that doesn't fit?" "Is it possible I have more than one problem?"

If your doctor doesn't have time for your questions and isn't capable of giving clear answers, find a better doctor.

Slow down the process. Studies have shown that physicians, on average, give their patients only eighteen seconds to tell their story before they interrupt. Yikes. You spend more time ordering a venti, extra-hot, sugar-free, five-shot, no-foam, pumpkin-spice latte at Starbucks.

If your doctor is distracted—interrupted by staff, looking at the clock or a computer—speak up.

"The inescapable truth is that good thinking takes time. Working in haste and cutting corners are the quickest routes to cognitive errors."

Beware of corrupt practices. It's well-known but still shocking: Some doctors get financial incentives or kickbacks to prescribe certain drugs or do suspect surgeries. "Spinal fusion may be the radical mastectomy of our time," Groopman writes.

Ask hard questions, and pursue second opinions. And please distrust any doctor who tries to turn the natural aging process into a disorder.

Every year, more than 250,000 Americans die from medical errors. You don't want to be one of them. It's a life-saving cliche: The best defense is a good offense. Find a doctor you trust and respect and can partner with. Be involved. Ask questions. Take a friend with you to take notes and listen.

And, finally, don't be intimidated by the white coat and framed medical degrees. Your doctor went to medical school. You didn't. But you've been thinking things through your whole life. Don't stop now. Start where you are. Learn what you need to know. And if she calls you by your first name, you do the same.

ENERGY EXPRESS-O! The Art of Medicine

"My doctor is wonderful. Once, when I couldn't afford an operation, he touched up the X-rays."
—Joey Bishop

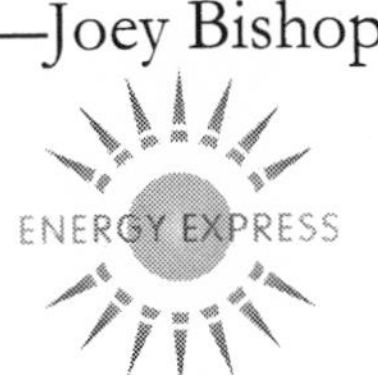

GOING DEEPER

If your doctor isn't willing to partner with you in the way Dr. Groopman describes, find one who is.

They are easier to find than they used to be. Do the research. Ask around, and look for key words to clue you in to a practice that combines the best of Western and Eastern practices: integrative medicine, complementary medicine, patient-centered medicine.

You want docs, nurses, physician assistants, therapists, nutritionists, and assorted practitioners who trained to take into account your whole being, a team who invites and encourages your involvement. You need them to be good listeners, not just prescription-writing machines. You can expect them to take the time it takes to make a proper diagnosis and then stay involved, with impeccable follow-through.

And find a doctor who doesn't see death as a failure, a doctor who isn't afraid to talk to you knowledgeably and compassionately about end-of-life issues.

Remember: The medical system in the U.S. is a for-profit business. It can be life-saving; it can be brilliant; but it is focused on treating illness, not preventing it. Your well-being depends on both, so don't settle for less.

I'm a real foodie when it comes to real food, and dining out in evolved, delicious, and conversation-friendly restaurants is one of the pleasures of my life. And then COVID-19 came, and everything changed. The good news? I became an even better and braver cook. Tens of thousands of restaurants closed, and thousands more opened up, and when we return to whatever passes for normal, I feel confident one thing will remain true: Eating out will still be a minefield. Portions are crushing. And food sources are suspect. How do I know my wild trout wasn't raised in a swimming pool? Join me in the sport of Menu Aerobics, an exercise in awareness for people with an appetite for knowing more and eating a little less.

Mind Your Menus.

For a long time, in the Before Time, dining out was our national pastime. So was porking up. Is there a link between the two? You bet your burgers. We're a fast-food nation of overeating eater-outers, and if you want to trim down and stay healthy, you might want to line up for personal instruction in one of my favorite sports: Menu Aerobics.

It's played sitting down, using your hands, with an assist from your nimble brain. The playing field is every restaurant on earth. The only skill you need is mindfulness. Eating out isn't the enemy. Spacing out is.

Split meals. When did portions in American restaurants explode? It's obscene. Europeans gasp at our supersize meals. Asians faint. We're one of the fattest nations in the world, with the heart disease and diabetes to prove it. And research supports the obvious: The more food on your plate, the more you eat.

So share an entree with someone else, preferably at your own table. Even if there's an annoying split-plate charge, it's worth it. More and more, smart restaurants are offering up half-orders or smaller portions. Train yourself to order less. Tell yourself you can always order more if you're still hungry. (You won't be.)

Focus on starters. Advanced players skip over the entrees. Instead, they focus on the appetizers, sides, and salads. That's where the gold is. The food's still a taste thrill; the portions are more manageable; and, yes, the prices are lower.

You'll also save hundreds of calories when you make a meal from two appetizers or one starter and a salad, but calorie counting isn't the point. It's not as irritating as texting at the table, but it can ruin the pleasure of the meal. When you eat, eat. Slow down. Chew. Savor every bite. Guilt around food is counterproductive, and it actually promotes indigestion.

Waist not, want not. Menu Aerobics is played best with a doggy bag. You order the entree you want, eat half, and take the rest home. If you meet a hungry person or stray animal on the way, bingo! If you resist taking leftovers because they tend to turn to pond scum at the back of the fridge, accept yourself as you are, and if no one else wants your half-portion of chicken tikka vindaloo, leave it on the table—with a nice tip for your server, just to help close the gap.

Skip over fried. Menu Aerobics gives you the core strength to glide quickly past the deep-fried stuff: the fried chicken, the fried fish, alas, the fried cheese balls.

It's not a matter of "bad" food as much as a bad habit. (Tasty, though.) When you have a lapse—and you will—and you wind up with a plate of fried onion rings the size of a chihuahua, at least pull off some of the breading.

This is extremely challenging in the case of crispy french fries, my weakness and my strength. I know I love them; I refuse to give them up. So I ask for the salt, count out nine beauties (not out loud), and hope to be conscious of every bite.

Then I move the rest out of reach.

(Full disclosure: I've been known to reach over three dinner plates to grab another handful of crispy fries, but please, do as I say, not as I do, unless you're willing to take responsibility for your actions. I am when it comes to fries, especially if I can get them with spicy Dijon mustard.)

Say the mantra. Memorize this phrase until it rolls off your tongue without the slightest embarrassment:

"Dressing on the side, please."

Was that so hard?

Practice at home, and repeat it with a smile in every restaurant you visit. I'm all for tasty sauces and dressings, but many places pour on way too much, and without thinking, you soak it all in.

Instead, dip your fork in, and sprinkle lightly.

Do you need bread? Some Menu Aerobic practitioners shun the buns and ask waiters to take the breadbasket away. Too many calories, too much gluten, too bloating. If you can't resist, satisfy yourself with a few bites or crusts. If you want butter—and who doesn't?—make a little go a long way.

Ordering wine? If you're not interested, fine, but if you are, savor every sip of the best wine you can afford, and exercise moderation. Then you can toast your good judgment, repeatedly, throughout the night.

Dessert! Talk about a minefield. Menu Aerobics doesn't require you to deny, deprive, punish. You already know that the healthiest dessert is fresh fruit, but there are genius pastry chefs out there determined to defeat your game plan. So, order one gorgeous caramel-coated brownie with two scoops of pecan green tea ice cream, and pass it around the table.

Take a bite; savor the pleasure, slowly; then say thank you, and kiss it goodbye.

ENERGY EXPRESS-O! Hold the Syrup

"I went to a restaurant that serves 'breakfast at any time.' So I ordered French toast during the Renaissance."
—Steven Wright

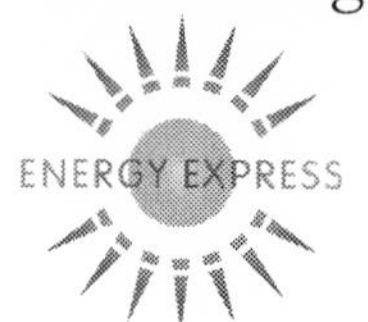

GOING DEEPER

Of course we want dining out back again. I do; you do; the whole restaurant industry is hungry for it to happen, the sooner, the better. What it will look like nobody knows. But here's one thing many people now know and consider another hidden blessing of COVID: Yes, eating out is fun, but cooking at home can be a total joyride, too.

And that's your challenge, if you choose to take it. Learn to cook and eat at home more often.

How will you make this happen? Trial and error? YouTube videos? Meal kits delivered to your house? The Food Channel?

Cooking tasty meals at home, using real ingredients and simple recipes, is as simple or complicated as you want to make it. It doesn't have to be time-consuming either. If there's a will, there's a way…so let me weigh in with this easy-as-pie idea.

This week, find a recipe for an entree that makes your heart sing, your mouth water. Caramelized onions under giant white beans with spinach and feta? Wild salmon with figs? Scrambled eggs with mushrooms and goat cheese? Figure out a few side dishes. Maybe a big salad, too.

Step two is to find some people to cook with. I realize COVID restrictions might still apply, so do the best you can until the time is right for people to gather again and share a kitchen.

What you prepare isn't nearly as important as the act of doing it, together.

And if you can get your kids into the kitchen to join you in food prep, on a regular basis, you'll earn frequent cooker miles and a permanent place in the Parenting Hall of Fame.

I keep a little pink Post-it note on my laptop, just to the left of the track pad. When it gets wrinkled and worn, I make a new one. It says, "Do The Practice." It's a reminder, an old-school version of the Apple watch that taps your wrist when it's time to stand up. Standing up is part of my practice. So is sitting still, doing yoga, race walking, nasal breathing, red wine, and making sure my boy Abraham gets enough playtime. So, what's your practice? If you don't have one yet, that's okay...But when you do, make a little note for yourself, and leave it where you can see it every day. It doesn't have to be pink.

Do the Practice.

Way before COVID, home gym spaces were getting big. You wake up and throw on what passes for workout clothes, and before you can find an excuse to skip it, you're walking on the treadmill or riding the stationary bike or pumping the weights and spreading joy throughout your body.

Yes! What could be better? No time-sucking commute to the gym. No monthly dues. No comparing yourself to the thinner and more buff all around you. (Never, ever do that.)

At home, it's just you and the practice and your growing awareness that regular exercise is the rock-solid foundation of a healthy lifestyle. You'll gain strength, reduce stress, and keep your joints juiced in a way that helps with agility and balance.

Exercising at home burns pounds of calories. But keep in mind: You can't outrun your fork. If weight loss is your goal, a home gym is a dear friend, but it's no substitute for smaller portions, a positive attitude, and a ban on processed foods and sugary cola drinks, especially the ones with fake sweeteners.

So make space, even if it's the corner of your bedroom or

a portion of the family room, and, need I mention, make it far from the fridge.

Make it inviting. Your workout space can be small, but if it's nasty—a dirty basement, a stuffy attic, a chilly garage—you'll find a reason to avoid it.

An area with natural light, fresh air, and no clutter is the feng shui ideal, but if that's not possible, start where you are. Make your space clean and appealing. A yoga mat and a fresh flower in your living room can work wonders on your mind and body. Whatever the size, treat it like the sacred space it is.

Feel good about what you spend. I don't know your budget for home gear, but two things I do know for sure: First, investing in your own wellness is money well spent. And second, don't buy cheap stuff. It will feel junky, and you won't use it. If you've got $5,000 or more to outfit an entire room, be thankful, but you can get just as fit for $500 or less, using free weights, stability balls, jump ropes, resistance bands, etc. It's easier than ever to find high-quality used gear—online, in specialty stores—but it's best to try it before you buy it, to make sure everything feels good and sturdy.

Plan for cardio, stretching, strengthening. For a balanced workout, your home gym should have at least one solid piece of aerobic equipment (a bike, a treadmill, an elliptical cross-trainer, your choice), plus space and gear for stretching and strengthening. If you're new to exercising, buy some time with a personal trainer (or consult with books, DVDs, etc.), and get started on a home routine that will safely deliver the results you want.

Make it user-friendly. Equip your space with whatever it takes to make your workout enjoyable. Music can be a great motivator. Exercise purists believe that watching TV or reading a book is a distraction. To get into the zone of peak performance, they advise you concentrate your attention on your inner body, your breathing. I know that's sound advice, but I also know how much I enjoy pedaling my recumbent bike while going through my magazine pile or talking back to the news shows.

Retreating to a workout space you've created mindfully—embellishing it with photos you love, stones you've kept, quotes that inspire you—will exert a powerful influence on your willingness to come back to it.

And don't forget to add a meditation cushion to the mix, even if you're not sure what to do with it. Someday, if you keep your brain healthy and curious, you'll sit down on it.

Keep a journal. To make the most of your home gym, show up every day. Keep a notebook, even if it's just a few lines. Jot down the date, what you did, and how you felt. If writing intimidates you, do it anyway.

Why? Keeping track in a journal is an ancient and highly effective magic trick when it comes to making change. It focuses you. It creates awareness. It will help you develop the habit of a regular exercise practice. I promise you that when that happens, your whole life will change in remarkable and delicious ways.

ENERGY EXPRESS-O! The Tao of Pooh

"A bear, however hard he tries, grows tubby without exercise."
—A.A. Milne

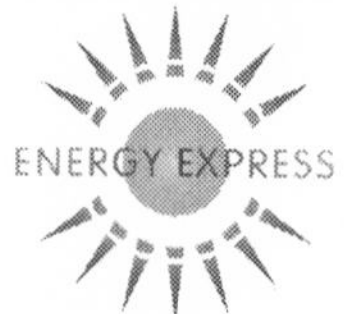

GOING DEEPER

Here's a question I hear a lot: When is the best time to do a home practice?

Is it early in the morning, when you're fresh and perky and want to wake up your body and mind to the whole day ahead of you?

Or is it later in the day, after work, after you've made a thousand little decisions and your body is desperate to unload some of the stress?

Here's the answer: The best time to do a home practice is when you will actually do it. It's a personal choice. When can you make time? When does it feel more like pleasure than punishment?

It may vary from day to day. That's okay, too. Some people use exercise to tire themselves out at night, to help them sleep. Others wouldn't dare jump on the treadmill after dinner because it gets the mojo going in a way that makes it harder to put it to bed.

There is no one best time to exercise. There is only the time that works best for you, this day, this moment. If it varies, let it vary. Just do the practice.

And if you miss a day, no sweat. Come back to it the next day. Begin. Again.

As your birthdays come and go, so might your interest in extreme rock climbing. It's okay to adjust our sports as we age. In fact, it's preferable if you want to have a sustainable practice, one that keeps your body strong and juicy, your mind calm and nurturing, all the years of your life. So let me introduce you to the idea of returning to a sport you once loved, now a better learner, now a slower-goer. The goal is to be a lifelong learner, adjusting when you have to so you can stay active, curious, and useful for as long as you can. When that's no longer possible? We want grace. As my friend Ana likes to say, "Walking, talking, dead."

Rediscover an Old Love.

I fell in love with the joy and thrills of cross-country skiing all over again on a recent backcountry holiday in the spectacular mountains of Pagosa Springs, Colorado.

The snow conditions were perfect; my companions were high-spirited; and I had the pleasure of re-learning a sport that is considered one of the greatest workouts there is.

I used to cross-country ski in the North Woods of Wisconsin, but then I moved to the Western mountains, and downhill skiing swept me off my feet. Repeatedly. Eventually, I gained new skills and became a solid intermediate skier with no interest whatsoever in going steeper, faster, bumpier.

"I like slow skiing," I used to tell my instructors, who never believed me. "I don't care about speed. I care about fun."

Learning to ski downhill gave me strength, confidence, balance, and edge control. It also gave me a concussion last year on an easy blue run: I slid headfirst into a rock, crushed my helmet, escaped a crippling injury—and decided in the emergency room to give cross-country skiing another go.

It was fabulous! No lines, no snowboarders, no $100 lift tickets. And no need for helmets. I'm not ready to ditch downhill, but I am inspired to tell you five things about cross-country skiing to encourage you to try it yourself:

It's an amazing workout. Downhill skiing won't develop your cardiovascular fitness; cross-country skiing will. You'll strengthen your heart and lungs, not to mention your legs, arms, shoulders, back, and core. Cross-country is a highly efficient aerobic sport, rhythmical and repetitive, requiring continuous effort, building endurance as you go. Downhill is a controlled fall down a mountain. In fact, if you want to downhill safely and well, you'll get in shape *before* you hit the slopes. And as a calorie-burner, cross-country beats downhill every step of the way. Every limb, every joint, is in motion, and you get the bonus of working your body in a cross-over fashion—right leg forward, left arm forward; left leg forward, right arm forward—that works both sides of your brain in a coordinated, balanced, blissful way.

Consider the cost. Cross-country skiing costs much less than downhill, so you can afford to do it more often. The best cross-country boots cost a third of what downhill boots cost, and they are a thousand times more comfortable. A day pass to use groomed trails might cost ten bucks compared to $40 to $100 or more to go downhill. And lessons! Learning to downhill ski can take years. You can absorb the basics of cross-country in a lesson or two and then practice, practice, practice. And then there's the cost of hurting yourself. Downhill skiing is considered a high-risk, high-injury sport. Cross-country isn't. The pace is slower, but the payoff can be just as thrilling.

It's fun for the whole family. I've heard it said that if you can walk, you can cross-country ski. It's not exactly true because there are skills involved, and you need to learn them to minimize your risk. But just about anyone can learn to cross-country ski, so the eight-year-olds and eighty-year-olds can play together, instead of just meeting for lunch.

The gear has improved. Backcountry cross-country skiing—ungroomed trails on wider skis, with edges—is giving new life to cross-country, and so is skate skiing. My new backcountry skis are much lighter (and shorter) than my old ones. It makes the uphills much easier and the downhills more controllable. Learning to snow plow is essential no matter what your gear, and the newer, lighter skis with edges make that much easier, too.

You connect to nature. When you downhill ski, you need to focus your full attention on your technique, your turns, and avoiding trouble. The margin for error is small. When you cross-country ski, not so much. It's slower, less risky, more meditative. You can look around, absorb the beauty, appreciate nature in all her winter splendor. Part of the magic of cross-country is the regular, repetitive breathing—slow, steady, deep. It takes you to another place, physically, mentally, spiritually.

I can't wait to go back.

ENERGY EXPRESS-O! Keep Smiling

"Cross-country skiing is great if you live in a small country."
—Steven Wright

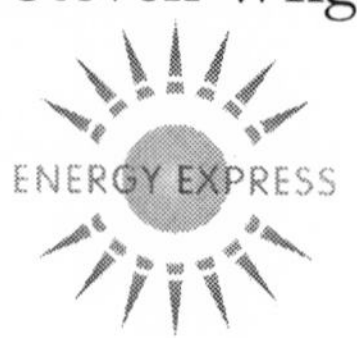

GOING DEEPER

If you can walk, you can cross-country ski. That's what I was told the first time I ventured out, and I believed it. Wrong. Cross-country skiing—one of the great workouts of the world—is a challenging aerobic sport. Don't expect it to come to you naturally. When you can relax into an understanding of the basics—the kick, the stride, the arm swing—you'll have more fun. And fun is why we play sports, right?

So, sign up for a cross-country lesson; rent the equipment; give it a try.

But resist giving it just *one* try.

If your body isn't used to the stride, the glide, the engaged core, the balance, it may rebel at first, screaming: "This is too hard. I can't do this. I want to stop!"

If and when that happens, shift away from the negative, and slow down. Way down. Take a few calming breaths, in and out of your nose.

Look around and notice how white the snow is, the brilliance of the sky, the sound your skis make when you press down on your forward leg.

Go back to your breath, listening to the sound of the inhale, the sound of the exhale, like the sound of the ocean, in and out of your nose.

Find pleasure in the rhythm, the flow: forward and backward, side to side, moment to moment.

You may find that cross-country skiing isn't your sport.

But then again, you may discover a new love.

One of the biggest threats to your well-being is the belief that the U.S. government is doing a decent job looking after your health and welfare. It is, in some ways, but in many more ways, it's not. At one point in the pandemic, America experienced greater numbers of COVID cases and more deaths than any other country in the world. Why is that? One reason is because we started off with so many millions of men, women, and children with compromised immune systems, obesity, asthma, heart and lung disease. And why is that? It's a complex and disappointing answer, and here's a big part of it: Our government is not doing what it could be doing to keep us safe from harmful foods and pesticides, toxic cosmetics and chemicals, polluted air, and yucky water. Capitalism invests in bottom-line profits, and there's a fortune to be made in ultra-processed foods and damaging personal care products, not to mention all the cancer-causing chemicals that make cleanup easier and health problems more likely. It's a deep, dark, overgrown jungle out there in Consumer Protection Land. And Roundup is oh, so not the answer. So, dear reader, until there is an answer...

Be Your Own Uncle Sam.

I've been on the healthy lifestyle beat for forty-five-plus years, and even though my readers sometimes scold me for being too political, I can't ignore the policies of health care. Well, I could, but it would be wrong.

Think about it: Your personal health and well-being is hugely influenced by public policy. The air you breathe, the additives in your food, the water you drink—or, increasingly, the water you can't drink anymore because it's no longer safe.

The people of Flint, Michigan, innocent victims of a national tragedy, were the canaries in the coalmine. And we all know it's not just Flint folks drinking impure, disease-causing water. All across America, red state, blue state, beleaguered health officials are in a state of panic and confusion over what to do to bring clean water to our cities and towns.

Our infrastructure is rotting beneath us, and citizens on the left, on the right, and straight up the middle are suffering. In 2021, it's still a pipe dream to think lawmakers will come together over clean water and clean air issues, but maybe they will. My question is: How could they not?

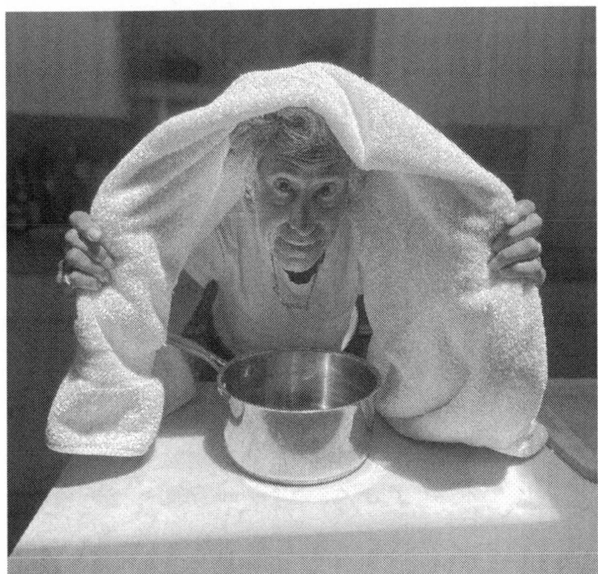

Moving on, it's been well-documented for too many years that there are poisons in our plastics and toxins in our toiletries. All of these are health threats to be reckoned with.

The U.S. government does its best—though I often wonder, best for whom?—but the best is not good enough when it comes to your personal well-being, dear readers.

Vigilance is called for—now more than ever because now is when we are dealing with the COVID-19 virus and all its variant cousins waiting in the wings.

Now is when we have to listen to the authorities, even when the authorities are confusing and, in some cases, thoroughly disgraced. If you want a clearer picture of what's happening, make an effort to listen and learn across the spectrum of advice, not just authorities from the right or authorities from the left.

In fact, for your well-being to prosper, you'll need to become your own authority on what you personally need to keep your immune system strong and resilient, your body nimble and energized, your brain as highly functional as the amount of distracting technology in your life will allow.

I call that Being Your Own Uncle Sam. It doesn't mean you give up on science or mainstream medical care. It means you listen with awareness, and you inform yourself about self-care and prevention, and you don't assume that every option offered by doctors and hospitals is what your body needs.

Remember when all the public health messaging was about eating no fat, low fat? Not only was it wrong, but it's pushed this country to dangerously high levels of obesity. Oops.

Remember bed rest for backaches? Another shameful screw-up by the medical authorities. Now we know that gentle movement is the way to go if you're ailing from a bad back, and really, who isn't ailing from a bad back these days?

Remember when sunscreen was supposed to save us all from skin cancer and medical authorities asked everyone, including babies, to wear as much sunscreen as possible and reapply often? The number of skin cancer cases didn't substantially reduce; in fact, it skyrocketed, as did the sales of sunscreen.

Remember the opioid crisis? One more horrifying example of what can happen when even good doctors do bad things to their patients, based on what Big Pharma told them was true.

I have file folders filled with more examples of government neglect, corporate malfeasance, and the collapse of our public health system, but instead, let me mosey on back to our tainted environment.

We've got decades of research and studies proving that manmade chemicals in our cosmetics, food, furniture, household cleaners, plastic bottles, toys, water—pretty much everything—are irrefutably linked to a hideously wide variety of cancers, heart disease, obesity, male infertility, and attention deficit disorders of all sorts.

"Of the more than 80,000 chemicals currently used in the United States," says the Natural Resources Defense Council, "most haven't been adequately tested for their effects on human health."

And how about this worthy-of-framing summary by the Environmental Defense Fund: "One of three formulated products sold by major retailers contains chemicals known to pose health risks."

Yikes. It's not just the FDA and the CDC that have fallen from grace since COVID. The underfunded, understaffed EPA hasn't been testing, and the chemical industry hasn't been resting, and we're all paying a sickening price when it comes to our national health and safety.

To be wary is to be wise. That's all I'm saying. That, and when will Congress come together and protect our collective well-being by passing strong and strict measures to ensure safe water, clean air, and foods that do no harm?

This shouldn't be political, right?

Am I crazy to think that evolved public health policies can become bipartisan policy? Yes, but it's the good kind of crazy.

Meanwhile, here is some more well-researched advice about Being Your Own Uncle Sam, from science reporter Alexandra Zissu.

(I admit that some of her suggestions sound a bit extreme. But so does the ever-increasing diagnosis of erectile disfunction.)

Turn up your nose at fragrances. Pretty smells can have ugly consequences, according to the research on a class of chemicals called phthalates, found in fragrances and countless consumer products.

Phthalates, even if you can't pronounce them, are endocrine disrupters. A few innocent sniffs and they're inside your body, mimicking hormones and creating havoc with your endocrine system, a network of hormones and glands that regulate everything you do.

So, check labels, and when in doubt, buy fragrance-free.

Think twice about plastics. Many plastics are carriers of hormone-disrupting chemicals that harm your health, even at very low doses. BPA is one of the bad-boy plastics to avoid…but how? Clean up your act one step at a time: Replace plastic food containers with glass ones; never use plastic in the microwave; replace plastic baggies with reusable lunch bags; and replace plastic cling wrap with beeswax-coated cloth. (I smile every time I cover half an apple with my reusable beeswax covers.)

Rethink kid cosmetics. Zissu reports that kids are using personal care products more than ever, and just like the adult kind, the kid-marketed cosmetics and lotions are packed with substances that get directly into the skin—the largest organ of the body—where they can do damage. Puberty, for instance, is coming on earlier than ever, and the complications aren't pretty. "Kids don't need cosmetics," Zissu reminds us. But the chemical industry always needs more customers, so that explains that.

Clean smarter. Don't get me started on household cleaners. Zissu suggests you dispose of the harsh chemical and toxic kind immediately! And responsibly, of course.

For more than forty years, we innocent zillions have been buying these big-bottle commercial cleaners—oven cleaners, flame retardants, chemical wipes—thinking they were harmless.

Summing up now, because this chapter is way too long for our shortened attention spans, our government isn't solving the devastating health problems our country is facing. In fact, it's helping to create them.

And no one is suffering more than the communities of color, where COVID hit hardest, took the most lives, and revealed a tragic misunderstanding of the social determinants of health.

That's why I end where I begin. Until something drastic happens in the way this country cares for its citizens, until we build back with a community-based, patient-centered, public health care system, the more important it is for you to Be Your Own Uncle Sam.

Seize the moment. Practice prevention. Engage in your own self-care, with respect for others and no guilt whatsoever for you. Don't be pressured or pushed into taking a drug just because the people behind the ad campaign want you to. Their job is to make money. Your job is to live a long and happy life.

ENERGY EXPRESS-O! Better Living Through Chemistry?

"Not everything that is faced can be changed, but nothing can be changed until it is faced."
—James Baldwin

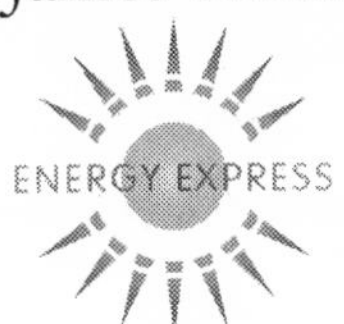

GOING DEEPER

If you can't trust the government to tell you what's safe and what's corporate greed and aggressive marketing, who can you trust? That's the trillion-dollar question. I don't have a good answer, especially now, with so much disinformation and misinformation competing for our lack of attention and messing with our minds. I will say, over the years, I've come to trust the facts and findings at www.EWG.org, a website run by the Environmental Working Group. If they one day go over to the dark side, please excuse me.

What foods should you buy organic? Which sunscreens are the most toxic? When will the government get phthalates out of our food supply?

The EWG labels itself a nonprofit, nonpartisan organization with more than twenty years of experience in pursuit of their mission: "to empower you with breakthrough research to make informed choices and live a healthy life in a healthy environment."

You'll find all sorts of useful information on the site, including the now famous "Dirty Dozen," a list of the fruits and vegetables you should buy organic because the conventional kind are so laden with harmful pesticides.

But wait. Shall we Go Deeper? It turns out even the Dirty Dozen list is being challenged by an opposing point of view. "The list was developed to invoke misplaced safety fears about fruits and vegetables," according to Safefruitsandveggies.com. The so-called Dirty Dozen list, they say, is "not scientifically supportable" and "may negatively impact consumers."

This nonprofit group wants you to eat more fruits and vegetables of every sort—organic and conventional—and it claims the Dirty Dozen list creates fear and paralysis and stops people from eating vegetables at all.

"If half of all Americans increased their consumption of fruits and vegetables by a single serving each day, 20,000 cancer cases could be prevented annually," they say.

That part is true, but as for the attack on the Dirty Dozen, who knows what's best for you?

You do, that's who! Be curious; do the research; make up your own mind...and please consume more real fruits and vegetables for the rest of your juicy and unspoiled life, accent on the juicy and unspoiled.

After my dear Papa Walter died in 1999, I found a little piece of paper folded up and tucked away in his wallet. He'd scribbled down little mottos that inspired him to be the tender and trusted man he was. "Do your giving while you're living, then you'll be knowing where it's going" is one I treasure. Another line he wrote down and I'm repeating often is, "Work smarter, not harder." Too much work brings on too much stress, and study after study has shown us that too much unrelieved stress makes us sicker, weaker, and more anxious, especially as we age.

Age With Attitude.

Aging isn't just for old people. We all do it. And many of us, witnessing our sagging skin, muddled brain, the dreaded chin whiskers, just don't like it.

That's because most people don't see it the way Frank Lloyd Wright did.

"The longer I live," this world-famous architect believed, "the more beautiful life becomes."

More mysterious, too.

"The secret to staying young," Lucille Ball revealed, "is to live honestly, eat slowly, and lie about your age."

There must be ten gazillion books on the subject of healthy aging. It's a multibillion-dollar industry that'll never die, even though every one of us will. That's why it's a compelling subject for all ages.

Instead of an overview, I'm going out on a limb to offer a point of view, my current nine rules—ideas? theories? self-delusions?—for healthy aging based on a lifetime of reading, writing, learning, exploring, and—oh, yeah—growing older.

Each rule could be a day's discussion or a twelve-week online course. Forget that. The clock is ticking; space is limited; and I want to keep it simple. In fact, keeping it simple is the tenth rule.

The order is random, much like life. Number one is not more important than number nine, unless it is to you:

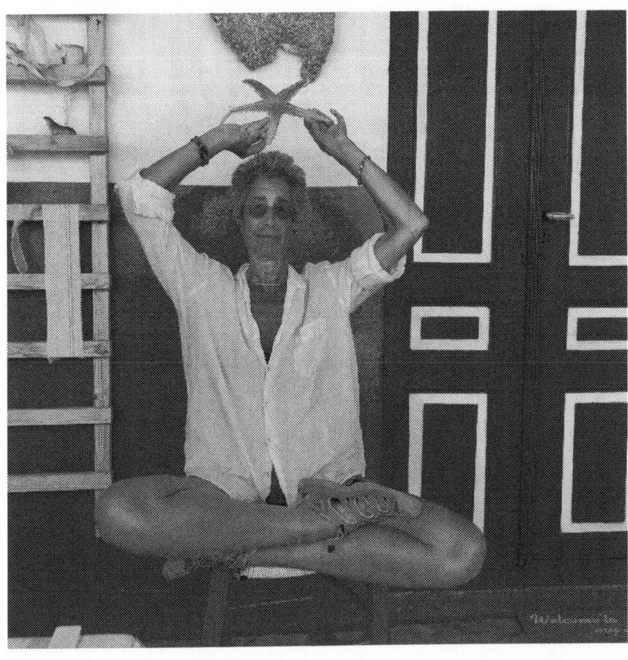

1. Expect success. Aging is not a disease. It's part of the natural flow of life. So embrace the positives about aging—wisdom and freedom are two biggies—and let go of the negative. People with positive perceptions of aging live seven years longer than people with negative perceptions. Their lives are not just longer, but happier, more meaningful. *Seven years longer!*

2. Exercise (mind and body). You can't hear this enough. To age gracefully, stay active. It's a must. Move it or it disappears. Walk, bike, swim, do yoga, whatever you like. Strength train, too. If you decide to run with only one of my so-called rules, make it this one.

3. Nourish your body. To age well, you have to eat well. That means real food, clean food, yummy food in amounts that don't make you sick or obese. The drama of dieting is over the day you give up processed foods, fake foods, sugary foods, and let the healthiest part of you prepare and eat food in reasonable portions that nourishes your body in a way that hot dogs and Pop-Tarts never will.

4. Accept what is. Strive to accept your life as it unfolds, without being angry or bitter or feeling victimized. At the same time, fight hard to live the best, most-balanced life possible. Don't dwell in the past or obsess about the future. Live in the moment, and respect, admire, and love the kind, compassionate person you are.

5. Rely on yourself. Self-care is the best care. Seek the finest medical care, but beware of overtreatment. Be smart about early detection and prevention, but avoid too much scrutiny. "What is a well person?" a doctor once asked his students. "A well person is a patient who hasn't been completely worked up."

6. Vent in healthy ways. Difficult things happen as you age. Sickness, pain, loss, not to mention the occasional global pandemic. You can't avoid the stress, but you can, you must, learn to deal with it in healthy ways. Yoga, Qigong, meditation, exist for that purpose. Find your own practice, your own path, and you'll know you're on it when your anger turns to forgiveness, your jealousy to joy.

7. Take risks. If you want to feel vital, fully alive as you age, keep taking risks. Keep challenging yourself. Keep testing your limits. "Go out on a limb," Jimmy Carter said. "That's where the fruit is." When was the last time you went out on a limb?

8. Do unto others. The older and crankier you get, the more kindness and forgiveness have to come into play. Helping others adds more meaning and purpose to life. Love and be loved, and you will live longer and die more gracefully. Most likely.

9. Understand death and dying. All that is living comes to an end. It's not if; it's when. So delve into it with humor, curiosity, and spirit. Find a community that supports your choices and beliefs. And remember this: No one on a deathbed ever says, "I wish I'd spent more time at the office."

Now, take the first letter for each rule—E-E-N-A-R-V-T-D-U—and play with the letters until you spell out a word that gets to the essence of healthy aging. Life's a great and mysterious game, and ultimately, just like aging, you have to unscramble it for yourself.

ENERGY EXPRESS-O! Everyone's an Expert

"The most important thing I can tell you about aging is this: If you really feel that you want to have an off-the-shoulder blouse and some big beads and thong sandals and a dirndl skirt and a magnolia in your hair, do it. Even if you're wrinkled."

—Maya Angelou

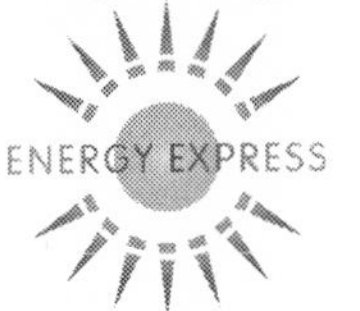

GOING DEEPER

Some time ago, way before COVID-19 but long after I knew I had no interest in ever coloring my hair, I was asked to give a keynote speech about aging. Thinking it over and over and over again, I came up with these nine rules.

It wasn't easy. My first draft had twenty-seven rules. It was a thirty-minute gig, so I did some heavy editing.

Now I'm happy I have them, and I'm asking you to do the same. Craft your own rules, that is.

What have you learned about life that you want to pass on?

What matters most? What turns out not to matter at all?

It's hard to pare a lifetime of experience down to nine oversimplified guidelines, but do it anyway, even if you're young.

It's an exercise in figuring out what you know now. Start where you are.

Here's one thing I know: What matters most at the end of your life is who you love and who loves you.

I forgot to mention it in my nine.

You'll forget stuff, too, so write down your nine rules and keep them tucked away on a piece of paper, revising as you evolve, scribbling down new truths as they come to you.

You never know who'll find it one day, maybe in your wallet, and put it to very good use.

The global pandemic forced us all to think out of the box, especially if you were sharing a small, smelly box with others. To think out of the box, we read great thinkers who shift our perspective and inspire our own creative thinking. Henry David Thoreau is certainly a role model for sparking our inner explorer. So are Seneca and Anne Lamott. Here are all three, with some superb advice about living your best, most authentic life.

Live a Big, Juicy Life.

My research shows that tens of millions of people make New Year's resolutions concerning their health. By the end of January, you can fit in a Fiat 500 all the people still on track, getting to the gym, walking the stairs, spending time on the cushion.

Relax. Finger-pointing and guilt-mongering, while still part of my cultural heritage, are wildly counterproductive when it comes to lasting lifestyle change. In fact, I have good news for you: Failing to stick to a resolution may not be your fault. It could be the resolution.

Maybe it's too shallow for you. You might do better latching on to a genius's resolution, one that takes you deeper and leads you to real growth and lasting transformation.

"At the start of each year, humanity sets to better itself as we resolve to eradicate our unhealthy habits and cultivate healthy ones," writes Maria Popova, on her splendid website, Brain Pickings (brainpickings.org).

Popova explains that while resolutions about better health are the most typical, "The most meaningful ones aim at a deeper kind of health through the refinement of our mental, spiritual and emotional habits—which often dictate our physical ones."

Here are three of my favorites from her list. If you see one you like more than "Zumba class twice a week," go for it. You've got nothing but time to make it stick:

"Walk and Be More Present."—Henry David Thoreau

It's one thing to tell yourself you'll walk more. It's a giant leap forward to challenge yourself to stay in the moment as you walk, without phoning or listening, without your mind straying to the past or future. How is that even possible? Focus on your breath and the sound of your breath. Feel the soles of your feet as you take every step. Why bother? Because, as Thoreau explained 150 years ago in an essay on the spiritual value of walking, walking without presence of mind is a missed opportunity to feed the soul and connect to your essential wildness.

"I am alarmed when it happens that I have walked a mile into the woods bodily, without getting there in spirit," he wrote.

Where's your spirit when you walk? To affect your deeper health, resolve to breathe in and out of your nose. If that means slowing down, slow down. Over time, you'll adapt, improve, thrive.

Be here now. I find this works just as well outside the woods.

"Make Your Life Wide Rather Than Long."—Seneca

"It is not that we have a short time to live," Seneca wrote about two thousand years ago, "but that we waste a lot of it."

Many of us coast through our lives, "in a trance of passivity and busyness—the greatest distractions from living," Popova writes, "mistaking the doing for the being."

Seneca agrees. In his treatise, "On The Shortness Of Life," he writes, "Putting things off is the biggest waste of life."

Don't squander your time, Seneca advises, because you never know how much you have. "The whole future lies in uncertainty: live immediately."

What if you resolved to "live immediately"? What are you putting off for later that would make your life richer and more satisfying right now?

"Let Go of Perfectionism."—Anne Lamott

"Perfectionism is the voice of the oppressor, the enemy of the people," Lamott writes in her classic *Bird by Bird* book about writing and life.

That inner voice telling you *you're* not good enough "will keep you very scared and restless your whole life if you do not awaken and fight back."

And how do you fight back? Make a lot of mistakes, she writes. Fall on your butt more often. And this: "Put something on your calendar that you know you'll be terrible at," Lamott advises, "like dance lessons, or a meditation retreat. Don't be so strung out on perfectionism and people pleasing that you forget to have a big juicy, creative life."

What if you resolved to have a bigger, juicier, more creative life this year? What would that look like?

Think about it. Don't let fear distract you. Want to play drums? Read in ancient Greek? Learn to paddleboard? Forget being perfect. Be forgiving to yourself instead, and see where enthusiasm, curiosity, and grace take you.

ENERGY EXPRESS-O! Let the Light In

"Ring the bells that still can ring
Forget your perfect offering
There is a crack in everything
That's how the light gets in."
—Leonard Cohen

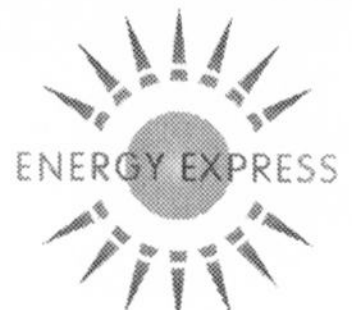

GOING DEEPER

To think out of the box, liberate yourself from your own excuses. Sign up for something you've always wanted to do but haven't so far because you always find a reason that gets in the way.

No time, no money, no one to go with, no way to get there…Just say no to all that, remembering that the mind attaches to the negative. That's the default. Pay no attention, and refocus on finding a way to live your dream, treating obstacles as crazy little annoyances to be overcome.

So, what'll it be? What would you do if you weren't afraid of failing or looking silly? Square dancing? Wall climbing? Pitching a tent in your own front yard?

And yes, please find a way to indulge yourself even in the aftermath of the global pandemic, because it's more important than ever ever ever to practice self-care. This is what gives you the strength to care for others. This is what makes caring for your well-being a sustainable practice.

Why wait?

Some say the jury is still out about the damage cell phone radiation is doing to our brains. That's because there is no real jury, not in the U.S., where cell phones have been judged as safe enough by the powers that be. And we are thankful that we have them, can't live without them, despite growing evidence that texting causes car crashes and radiation overexposure is damaging and young brains are being rewired in ways that put them at risk. Let's face (time) it: Unending distraction is the new normal, and smartphones aren't going away. So, what do we do? We become aware. We resist the addiction. We double down on self-care. We use the off button.

Outsmart Your Smartphone.

I know I'm sticking my neck out, but it's high time we take a deeper look at what technology is doing to our bodies as we spend hours and hours, day after day, year after year, looking down at our phones, our screens, and, now, our politicians.

Talk about shaping your destiny. The medical malady cutely called "text neck" is on the rise as we conduct our COVID-impacted lives more and more on mobile devices—head forward, neck compressed, eyes lowered, shoulders slumped.

It may look harmless, but it's not. Over time, this downward-looking posture has unintended and very expensive health care consequences. (This is more than a hunch.)

The spine gets stressed; the discs get compromised; and your kids walk with their heads so far forward their noses are ahead of their toeses. Here are just a few of the problems we suffer when we let our devices take a toll on our anatomy

Neck pain, shoulder pain, back pain, leg pain, foot pain.

Chronic headaches and arthritis.

Pinched nerves and herniated discs.

Feelings of powerlessness and anxiety.

And that's not all.

"Think ADHD, immune issues, allergies, fatigue, and hormone imbalances," says Dr. Matt Thompson, a chiropractor based in Highlands Ranch, Colorado. He is alarmed at what he's been seeing. So am I. So should we all be.

"The advent and abundance of technology is skyrocketing 'forward head posture' and 'text neck' in the U.S. and worldwide," he said.

"Practically, this means any signal between brain and body, both function and feeling, can be affected."

Any signal between brain and body?! That can't be good.

And it gets worse.

"Maintaining this forward head posture…stimulates the primitive brain while neglecting the higher brain," explained Dr. Thompson. "This creates an immature brain balance between the left and right hemispheres, which can lead to behavioral, social, and immune system issues."

Oh dear. Behavioral, social, and immune system issues all take a toll on your well-being. But you know that, right?

Heavy is the head. The average adult head weighs between ten and twelve pounds, depending on whether or not you were drinking the night before.

"For every inch the head goes forward beyond the shoulder, this is ten to fifteen extra pounds of stress and tension on the entire spine," says Dr. Thompson. He's talking about maybe sixty pounds hanging off your fragile neck, just so you can see the Instagram post of your friend's cat wearing a Cubs hat. "This can create pain, fatigue, soreness, headaches, vision and attention problems."

Text neck pressures your cervical spine. Text neck, over time, can take the natural curve out of your neck, straighten your cervical spine, stretch the spinal cord, and put pressure on your brainstem.

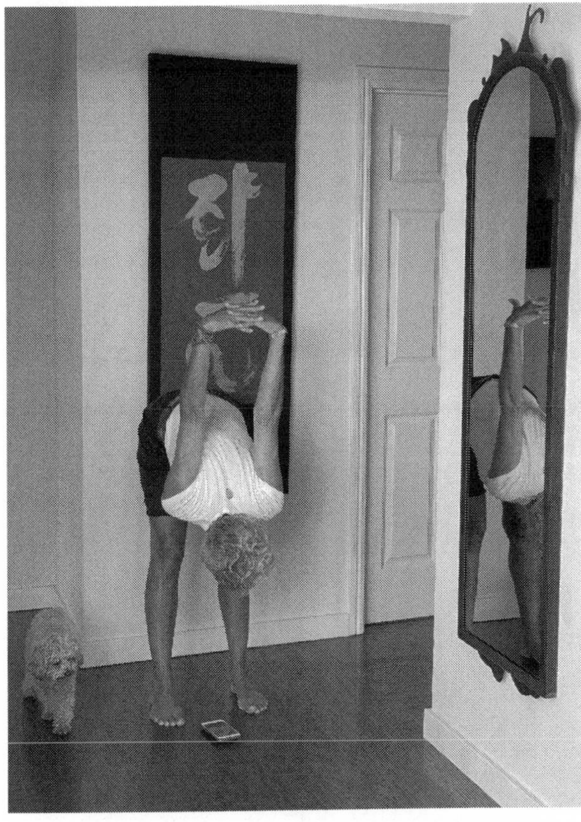

This is what sickness feels like, followed by pain, followed by millions of prescriptions for painkillers, which don't work well and tend to be addictive.

You're all connected. The slumped, looking-down-all-the-time posture isn't just bad for the body. It's also a big drag on your emotions, your spirit, your sense of power. That's the conclusion of many scientists, including social psychologist Amy Cuddy, associate professor at Harvard Business School.

She's the bestselling author of *Presence* and presenter of a sensational 2012 TEDGlobal talk seen by over 62 million viewers.

As we know, the mind and body are connected. And so, Dr. Cuddy reports, when your body slumps, so do you, in subtle and debilitating ways. The text-neck pose—blocking our energy, straining our muscles—creates feelings of powerlessness and anxiety.

All this plus pain, fatigue, and brain fog.

Okay, it's time for a serious heads-up.

Prevent text neck before it takes a toll. There are things you can do—besides quitting your job to bake bread in a Zen monastery—that can help you lower the boom on text neck and maybe prevent it.

—Read your screens at eye-level. Selfie sticks are useful, and so are adjustable device holders, easily found online. For desk work, get and please use a stand-up desk. For those times when you're out and about, just use your perfectly placed arms.

—Team up with savvy practitioners who specialize in the analysis and correction of spinal posture and speak the language of prevention.

—Take breaks; do stretches; train in a mind-body awareness practice such as yoga, Qigong, the Alexander Technique, Feldenkrais, or somatics so you can sense building tension before it explodes into chronic pain.

—And this, dear readers: If you want to feel and act persuasively and authentically, rise up from your habitual screen slouch, and follow Dr. Cuddy's advice, strike the Power Pose—head up, eyes forward, shoulders wide, hands on hips, legs spread.

Ain't no body gonna mess with you.

ENERGY EXPRESS-O! Authenticity 'R' Us

"Let your body tell you you're powerful and deserving,
and you become more present, enthusiastic,
and authentically yourself."
—Amy Cuddy

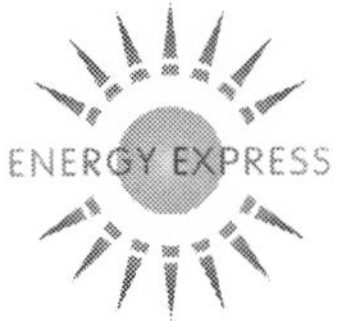

GOING DEEPER

The Power Pose—also known as the Wonder Woman pose—is something to try when you're feeling COVID distress or stress of any kind. For many of us, that's about eighty percent of our day.

It involves standing tall, hands on hips, chest open, head positioned comfortably over your spine. A slight smile on your face is optional, but I recommend it. Don't be shy about trying it and seeing how it feels. How it feels is the point.

This Wonder Woman pose works equally well for all genders, but it's especially empowering for girls and women, who often need empowering the most.

And how exactly does it work? Amy Cuddy, among others, has proven that your body language impacts the level of testosterone and cortisol in your body. Striking the Power Pose raises your testosterone and lowers your cortisol.

Higher testosterone levels—in females and males—lead to greater confidence. Lower levels of cortisol make you feel less anxious and more able to deal with stress.

Wonder Woman positions you to be more assertive, more willing to take risks, more relaxed. It's the ideal thing to do every day—before school, an important meeting, a confrontation with a workplace creep.

You are how you stand. Strike this pose for two minutes a day for a couple of weeks, and zone in on how it makes you feel, inside, where only you can focus. Consider the following variation to make it even more effective:

While standing in the pose, close your eyes or gaze softly into the middle distance. And try this simple nasal breathing exercise: Breathe in deeply for a count of four; hold for two; and then breathe out slowly, through your nose, to a count of five.

Pause after, and wonder about this: How does your body feel after the Power Pose? Can you tune in to sensation, pulsations, emotions? Go deeper. Do you feel calmer? More spacious in that tender area behind your heart?

Arrange your facial muscles into a serene smile, even if you have to use your hands.

Does the smile shift how you feel? Of course it does. It's the embodiment of All Is Well.

"It's not that I'm afraid to die. I just don't want to be there when it happens." I still laugh whenever I hear that old Woody Allen joke, but my thinking about death and dying has evolved over the years, thanks to decades of living with the consequences. I was there when my mother died. I was there when my father died. And I want to be there when I die. Arranging that in a society hell-bent on turning dying into a problem to be solved isn't easy, but it's more and more possible. If you've ever been involved in end-of-life care, you know what a blessing hospice and palliative care can be. To me, it's one of the best developments in modern medicine in the last forty years. So is the medical, recreational, and scientific use of cannabis, but now I'm way off topic. So, have you thought about where you want to die? In a hospital...or at home? In a nursing home or in hospice? I know it's not something you want to think about right now, or ever, but believe me, when you do put a plan in place, your personal well-being will take on a heavenly glow.

Start the Conversation.

Have you had the Conversation?

Probably not. Most people don't until it's too late.

However, more people are having it now, since COVID. It actually feels good to have that Conversation, once you get started. But getting started can be tricky.

I began the Conversation in the kitchen of my niece's house some years ago. A ninety-one-year-old elder we both knew had died, and I found myself saying that the way Dorris died—in her bed, surrounded by loving family and friends, no fear, no pain, touched and held until the end—was a blessing, not only in her life but in mine, too. It inspired me to cue the harps and face the music when it comes to thinking about, and planning for, my own final breath.

And that's what the Conversation is—an honest and open discussion with your loved ones about what you do want and what you do *not* want when it comes to end-of-life care.

The Conversation isn't necessarily a one-time event. It will evolve as you do: Home care or hospital? The Beatles or Bach? Candles or cannabis or both?

The end-of-life Conversation is personal and private, but it needs to happen while you're healthy, because when the time comes to really spell out the details, it might be too late.

"It's always too soon until it's too late," writes Ellen Goodman, the Pulitzer Prize-winning journalist who co-founded The Conversation Project, a "public engagement campaign with a goal that is both simple and transformative: to have every person's end-of-life wishes expressed and reported."

What a divine idea!

"It's not surprising that we postpone and postpone these conversations. Talking about dying is hard," Goodman says. "When I opened the subject with my own daughter Katie, her first response was 'Can't we just have lunch?'" Goodman isn't joking when she writes and speaks about the heart-wrenching experience of her mother's death and the enormous gap between what people say they want at the end of life and what actually happens.

Here are some eye-opening statistics from The Conversation Project, in collaboration with the Institute for HealthCare Improvement:

—Seventy percent of people say they prefer to die at home…but in fact, seventy percent of people die in a hospital, nursing home, or long-term care facility.

—Eighty percent of people say if seriously ill, they would want to talk to their doctor about end-of-life care…but in fact, only seven percent report having had end-of-life conversations with their doctor.

—Ninety percent of Americans know they should have a conversation about what they want at the end of life…yet only thirty percent have done so.

If so many people want to have the Conversation, why isn't it happening?

One reason, according to The Conversation Project survey, is that people simply don't know how to get it going.

Imagine a family gathering. It's Thanksgiving, the perfect time to be grateful for the life you have and the end-of-life care you want. But how do you pause the football game and begin? What do you say?

And that's where The Conversation Project's end-of-life starter kit comes into play. It's a free download from their website, a well-written, step-by-step guide that gives you tools, medical directives, resources, and more than a few questions to get the Conversation going.

Here, for instance, are some questions a son or daughter might ask an aging parent before he or she gets a diagnosis, before they end up in intensive care:

"When you think about the last phase of your life, what's most important to you?"

"When would it be okay to shift from a focus on curative care to a focus on comfort care?"

"On a scale of one to five, with one being, 'I want to live as long as possible, no matter what' and five being, 'Quality of life is more important to me than quantity,' where do you stand?"

"We want you to be the expert on your wishes and those of your loved ones," The Conversation Project makes clear. "Not the doctors or nurses. Not the end-of-life experts. You."

The starter kit gets you talking, and just as crucially, it gets you listening.

Listen to what your spouse wants, your brother, your best friend. Listen without judging. Just listen. And listen to your own answers when you're having the Conversation. The more you talk through the details of your own end-of-life care, the better you'll feel.

That's been my experience, beginning in my niece's kitchen that day, and I'd bet my life it'll be true for you.

"This isn't about dying," the experts say about having the Conversation. "It's about figuring out how you want to live till the very end."

ENERGY EXPRESS-O! You Be the Decider

"In being with dying, we arrive at a natural crucible of what it means to love and be loved. And we can ask ourselves this: Knowing that death is inevitable, what is most precious today?"

—Joan Halifax

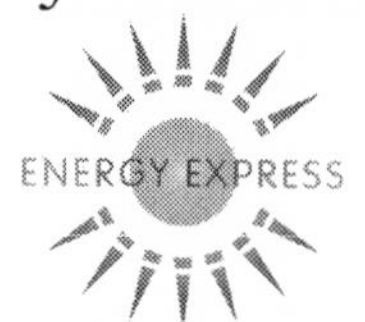

GOING DEEPER

Dr. Atul Gawande—the influential writer, surgeon, and health care reform advocate—has written a magnificent book about death and dying called *Being Mortal.*

It's a bestseller with a cult following, and one surprising truth it reveals is that doctors in America are taught to see death as a failure.

It reminds you, dear reader, to take end-of-life matters into your own hands, your own heart, if you want to exit with grace and gratitude.

"You don't have to spend much time with the elderly or those with terminal illness to see how often medicine fails the people it is supposed to help," Gawande writes. "The waning days of our lives are given over to treatments that addle our brains and sap our bodies for a sliver's chance of benefit."

As soon as I finished reading *Being Mortal*, I started it again. And then I bought a copy for many in my family, and then my friends, and then I told strangers on airplanes to read it, and now…you. It's that good.

Another brilliant book to help you go deeper into dying was written by my friend Roshi Joan Halifax, founder of the Upaya Institute and Zen Center. It's called *Being With Dying: Cultivating Compassion and Fearlessness in the Presence of Death*, a classic published in 2009 and now the foundation of a training program taught in hundreds of medical and educational institutions around the world.

We all want a "good death," but the truth is we're going to get the death we get, Roshi Joan teaches.

So, how do we make the most of that death, without judging, without suffering to extremes, with clarity and acceptance and love?

Those are the final questions in this, the final chapter of the book. Even if you don't feel like flipping it over and starting again, I'm grateful for your attention, now and forever.

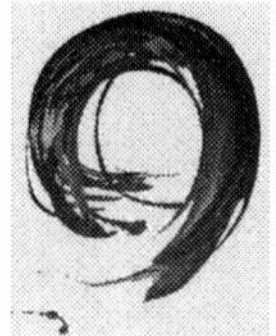

Afterword.

In the middle of March, I had to stop doing research and rewrites for the second edition of *All Is Well* and put this baby to bed.

It was hard to stop fussing and fixing, because every day in early 2021 brought new developments in the COVID crisis: more economic stress and personal struggles; more about vaccines and variants; many more decisions to be made affecting your own personal well-being.

Here were the headlines in The New York Times on March 15, 2021, the day I decided to put this second edition on lockdown:

—*Germany and France become latest to suspend use of AstraZeneca vaccine.*

—*Italy imposes lockdown measures as cases spike in Europe.*

—*A year into the pandemic, parents are demanding that schools fully reopen.*

—*Millions have left the labor force, many home with children or health concerns.*

—*Mental health crisis affecting young people needs immediate attention, report says.*

I'll stop now. As COVID continues—we'll be feeling the aftershocks for years—who can say what will happen next?

"The only thing we can be sure of is that we can't be sure of anything," my wise Greek friend Athena told me on the phone this morning, just before I pulled the trigger on booking my ticket back to Greece for late May 2021.

I'm writing this Afterword on March 15.

"Beware the Ides of March."

Really? That's what Shakespeare told us in *Julius Caesar.* And for hundreds of years since, the fifteenth of March has been synonymous with disaster, tragedy, warnings ignored.

That's not how I see things this March 15, 2021, in spite of the grief and suffering all around. Everything changes. COVID will pass, and future health scares will come and go, and the question from me to you is: What can you do to prepare, prevent, prevail?

The global pandemic has been labeled by many as an apocalyptic event. In Greek, the word apocalypse doesn't mean the end of the world, as people assume. It doesn't mean doom and gloom, the end of times, a cosmic kaput. In fact, the Book of Revelations has a happy ending.

The word apocalypse comes from the Greek word "*apocalupsis,*" meaning unveiling, uncovering, a revelation of great knowledge that was hidden before.

It's a derivative of the verb "*apokalyplein,*" to take the cover off.

The COVID pandemic blew the cover off a world that had grown complacent and cruel, unjust and unhealthy for so many.

But don't beware this ides of March. *Be aware.* What did COVID reveal to you that you didn't know before?

Please don't shut down, go numb, live in fear, in negativity, waiting for the next horrible news headline to grab your attention and crush your spirit.

Instead, find yourself on the path of awareness, starting with self-awareness. Be more aware than you have ever been, and let the light of that awareness lead you to your own path to a better life and an easier death, greater health and happiness, and whatever else you need to live that one wild and precious life of yours.

Be aware that neuroscience reveals that the mind attaches to the negative, and there's still a big, bright, beautiful world out there—filled with opportunity, love, and grace—waiting for you to explore.

Be aware that your inner world is every bit as big as the world out there. Be curious about ways to explore it, too. Slowing down will help. So will yoga, but my sister's already made me aware that yoga isn't for everyone and I shouldn't be talking about it so much. She's right. And still…

Be most aware of this: that even if the medical authorities don't tell you to boost your own immune system, do it anyway. Become your own medical authority. Have an intentional self-care practice. All your efforts will be rewarded. Move your body every day. Get plenty of sleep. Eat real food. Be grateful. Help others. Stay close to people you love and people who love you.

Is all that an absolute guarantee you won't get COVID or any one of its deadly variants? No. There are no 100% guarantees…except that one final breath that guarantees your time as an Earthling is over.

Be aware that the ability to adapt and survive is in your DNA, and you are uniquely qualified to make decisions that are right for you. So don't be pushed or pulled onto a path that isn't your own.

Or else—beware!—your personal well-being will rise up and bite you on the ass.

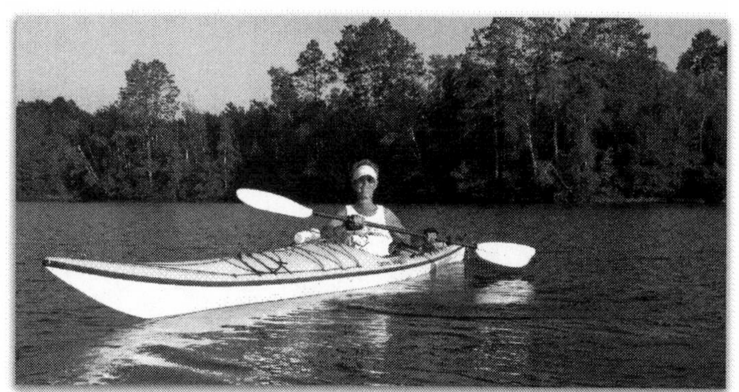

Acknowledgements.

Let me close with deep bows to Creators Publishing—led by Rick Newcombe and his son, Jack Newcombe—with a special shout-out to my editor for the first edition, Simone Slykhous.

They inspired and encouraged me to write *All Is Well,* published in 2017, and in June 2021, a new creative team at Creators stepped in to launch this second edition.

Thank you, Kelly Evans and Alessandra Caruso, for your talent, your enthusiasm, and everything you've done to make this new edition bigger, bolder, better. Thanks also to Samantha Peloquin and Alex Nagy of the Creators team.

I wholeheartedly acknowledge and applaud all the help and guidance I've gotten from the creative team at BadDog Design, especially founder and alpha female, Peggy Pfeiffer, as well as Antonio Cassidy.

Peggy, who designed the covers of both editions, convinced me I needed a better website and some kind of presence on social media, and she helped me get there in spite of my pathological resistance to posting and pushing. I keep reminding her I have an analog brain in a digital world, and I'm grateful she understands.

It was Peggy's wonderful idea to feature Kaz Tanahashi's striking enso of imperfection on the cover, and I thank Kaz for saying yes.

I also want to express boundless gratitude to my unconditionally loving parents, Walter and Marcia, my remarkable sister Charna, my entire, ever-expanding family, every dear friend, every teacher, every interview, every training, every book I've read and yoga class I've taken.

And yes, thank you to the intrepid husband I rode bicycles in France with and was married to for thirty-five years.

All of them and all of it enabled me to discover, cherish, and not shy from the path to my own well-being.

And who more than Barbara? My adored editor-in-chief, who introduced me to the bliss of eating crispy fries, riding bikes that are really our ponies, and trusting the sea even when you can't see to the bottom.

We married in 2014, on the spring equinox. She died June 11, 2019, and I dedicate this second edition to her. Sweet dreams, darling one.

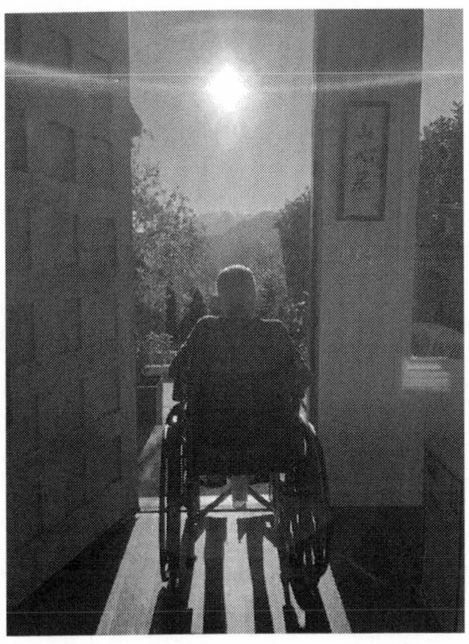

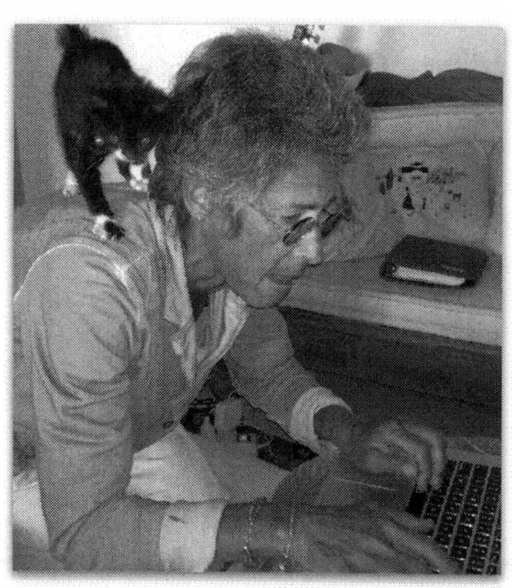

About the Author.

Marilynn Preston—acclaimed journalist, healthy lifestyle expert, Emmy-winning TV producer—is the author of the Amazon bestseller, *All Is Well: The Art {And Science} of Personal Well-Being.*

All Is Well is based on her forty-plus years writing "Energy Express," America's longest-running syndicated fitness column. "Energy Express" ran in dozens of newspapers all over the country for forty-three years, and in May 2019, Marilynn ended the column and, with much-appreciated tech support, continued to post on MarilynnPreston.com, Instagram, and Facebook.

Marilynn has written two other books, *Dear Dr. Jock: The People's Guide To Sports and Fitness* and *Work Well, Be Well.* She also created, exec produced, and co-wrote the nationally syndicated "Energy Express" TV series about sports, fitness, and adventure for kids and families. For this work, her team won two Emmys and a Women's Sports Foundation award for outstanding programming. EN/X ran in 120 cities while it lasted and lives today as a vintage YouTube channel.

Marilynn is the founding chair of a life-changing nonprofit called Girls in the Game, based in her hometown of Chicago. More than twenty-five years after GIG began, she still works as a shameless and enthusiastic board member, helping girls get the healthy lifestyle training they need to become strong, confident, powerful women.

Please visit www.girlsinthegame.org to meet the girls, hear their stories, and make a donation to the Self Care Project (support.girlsinthegame.org/campaign/teens-self- care-project/c342954), where girls get coached in movement and meditation, self-acceptance, journaling, resiliency, and many more life-affirming self-care practices celebrated in *All Is Well.*

Marilynn's own practice—in case you're curious—includes slow yoga, meditation, race walking, kayaking, cycling, nasal breathing, wine tasting, and as much adventure travel as she can fit in. She's circumambulated Mount Kailash in Tibet, climbed Mount Olympus in Greece, bicycled in France and Italy, golfed in Bhutan, and scuba dived in the YMCA pool in Chicago.

Her next big adventure is getting people to read and enjoy the second edition of *All Is Well*—the COVID edition—to create their juiciest, most joyful lives.

All Is Well

The Art {and Science} of Personal Well-Being
2nd Edition
The Covid Edition, 2022
is also available as an e-book for Kindle,
Amazon Fire, iPad, Nook, and Android e-readers.
Visit creatorspublishing.com to learn more.

° ° °

CREATORS PUBLISHING
737 3RD ST.
HERMOSA BEACH, CA
310-337-7003

° ° °

Made in the USA
Middletown, DE
27 February 2023